MW00744354

Margaret Gilbeth

SILVER LININGS

Living with Cancer

Margaret Chrislock Gilseth

Ye fearful saints, fresh courage take
The clouds ye so much dread
Are big with mercy, and will break
With blessings on your head.
—William Cowper

VANTAGE PRESS
New York

FIRST EDITION

Published by Vantage Press, Inc.
516 West 34th Street, New York, New York 10001

Manufactured in the United States of America
ISBN: 0-533-11253-2

Library of Congress Catalog Card No.: 94-90476

0 9 8 7 6 5 4 3 2 1

To my caring husband
Walter,
strength at my side.

Contents

Foreword

What do faith, love, and joy have to do with staying alive? According to Margaret Gilseth, everything. This true account of one woman's courageous commitment to living with cancer despite all odds spans thirty-seven years, as she faced several major life-threatening surgical procedures.

She recounts the fear and the pain, but far more memorable is her commitment to live. Rather than become a useless invalid or die, Margaret places her life in the hands of God and takes advantage of every opportunity to experience a full and satisfying future. With her husband and son, she moves from Washington State to Africa on a teaching mission. While there she is sent from Nairobi, Kenya, to a hospital in London for radiation therapy. Later she and her husband travel to Mexico, Nicaragua, and back to Africa with a team of optometrists distributing eyeglasses in the Third World. Relating each encounter, she offers us a unique insight into her surroundings as well as the people she meets.

This is a sensitive, often humorous message to cancer sufferers. Equally important, however, while *Silver Linings* describes her long battle against cancer, its message speaks to all of us who, for one reason or another, allow the mystical beauty of life to pass us by, afraid of what tomorrow might bring. For Margaret, she simply doesn't have time for fear.

Theresa Gervais Haynes
Albuquerque, New Mexico

SILVER LININGS

1

April 4, 1957, the Diagnosis

They cut away her breast! Amputation! I was stricken by what was happening to our pastor's wife, a dear, good friend. I was twenty-five at the time and knowledgeable to a degree about breast surgery, called by the less startling term, radical mastectomy. My father died of a cancer that began with a lump found in his chest. My mother died suddenly after colon surgery. I knew about cancer.

They said my friend would have a swollen arm, perhaps indefinitely. Would the cancer recur? There was no way of knowing: one would simply have to live with that more than likely development. Her daughter said she didn't sleep well at night and kept an aspirin bottle beside her bed. As I look back on this sudden rush of dread, I wonder whether it was an omen, a foreshadowing of things to come.

I had just passed my thirty-eighth birthday when cancer's ugly curse descended on me. I taught English at the public high school in Lynden, Washington, where we lived. My husband, Walter, taught in a school twenty miles away. We had one son, Steven, who was six, and two foster children, Ron, seventeen, and his sister, Carolyn, fifteen. We were settled in our respective classrooms with an established routine until . . .

I discovered the lump in my breast as I lay in bed one Saturday morning reluctant to begin the day. I lay on my right side, my left breast resting on my right, when I felt a small lump the size of a kidney bean. Had I been searching for something? Hardly, but I almost thought so. Dismissing it as a cyst, I decided to have the doctor look at it—sometime.

The time came the following week when our son had eczema flare up behind his knees. He returned from the doctor with a jar of salve and I with a hospital appointment. "We cannot put this off," our family doctor said with all seriousness. "It could be just a benign cyst, but we must be on the safe side."

I entered St. Joseph Hospital in Bellingham at three o'clock in the afternoon of April 4, 1957, into a room with its only window obstructed by a concrete bulkhead. Since surgery wasn't scheduled until eight the next morning, I brought along a copy of *King Lear,* intending to fill the interim with catch-up reading for a unit on Shakespeare I was teaching to a class of seniors. I felt awkward going to bed in the middle of the afternoon, but that was the procedure and I knew better than to protest. It proved conducive to reading, however, for there were few interruptions.

The forsaken old king, lost in a storm, spoke to me:

> Expose thyself to feel what wretches feel,
> That thou mayst shake the superflux to them,
> And show the heavens more just.

Certainly profound words on being myself at the brink of upheaval, I thought, as I set the book aside and slid between crisp sheets on the high, firm bed.

A nurse entered with medications. "A pill for sleeping," she said, smiling cheerily.

"I hardly think I need one," I replied with assurance.

"All the same, I would take it." She spoke with authority now. I swallowed the pills. Tomorrow I would know whether more than a cyst was embedded in my breast. The lights were lowered and I slept.

My fear returned the next morning as I received a shot of Demerol rather than breakfast. At the same time a cart clattered in, and I was wrapped well in blankets and hustled onto it.

The operating room was cold and metallic. Fluorescent lights beamed with startling whiteness. Several doctors and nurses, white as the light, grinned greetings at me, which I scarcely acknowledged.

The anesthesia brought Wagner's prelude to the first act of *Lohengrin.* I experienced dimension, unfathomable distance! Piercing violins pinned a speck in the sky. How close would it come? In the music, I remembered, it drew nearer until it became the Holy Grail. Would it now? Or would it diminish into nothingness?

My husband, Walter, was called out of the waiting room into a small room next to the operating theater, followed by a surgeon who was wearing bloodstained operating garb. Two others followed.

"Your wife's tumor is malignant." The first doctor removed his face mask and spoke respectfully. "We removed it, but we need to go further."

"Go further?"

"Yes, which means doing a radical—going under the arm. Because we do not want it to spread to the lymph nodes, we recommend this procedure."

A second doctor stepped forward. "It means that your wife's prognosis is good because she came to us early."

"We need your consent to proceed," continued the first. "She is still under anesthesia, and we are prepared to carry on."

Walt looked from one to the other. "If that is what you recommend, so be it."

("I had to face up to this while you were still on the table," Walt told me later.)

I must have been moved, for there was a chrome light fixture in the ceiling. High vibrant violins still twitched—I felt as well as heard them, even inhaled them. I came from far away, not falling like Alice in Wonderland exactly, nor moving with perfect control like a bird, just floating. I opened my eyes again. I was back in my room as I recognized the window with the bulkhead obstructing the sunlight. I needed sunlight. Consciousness was returning.

"I see you're waking up," said a voice.

So I am waking up after anesthesia, I thought, as I turned my head toward the voice. With effort I focused my eyes and recognized my surgeon.

"You're awake," he repeated, taking my hand.

I acknowledged him, but Wagner's violins were too loud for me to fully realize why he was there. He had come to tell me cancer had been found. But it would not be my cancer, not mine. . . .

I focused again. His eyes told me what he had to say. *Why am I not seized with panic? I must indeed be brave. Bravo!* I sank back among the violins.

During my next encounter with consciousness, I tried frantically to free myself from the weights that clung to my limbs. In so doing, I discovered I was between crisp sheets again and, oddly, with a pillow under my head.

Suddenly a surge of pain and overwhelming fatigue stabbed without warning through my left shoulder. *My breast is gone! I have a terrible wound! Excruciating pain!*

Several nurses surrounded me. "We will give you something for your pain very soon." said one. "We only need to know you are awake."

A shot in the hip and I sank again. No violins this time—what I inhaled was fresher. The silence was a blessing!

Paper rustled, "Flowers for Mrs. Gilseth," said a happy voice.

"Who from?" I actually exclaimed like a child.

"It says here, Senior Class," came the reply. "How beautiful! We'll put them in a vase right away."

Immediately I saw my classroom and all the familiar faces. How thoughtful, how kind! A surge of emotion—flowers, how special I felt!

"Your husband is here," the happy voice spoke again. "He's waited for you all afternoon."

He couldn't have. It was still morning, wasn't it? Then I realized the room was artificially lighted. Last evening I had been reading; the book was in the drawer of the bedside stand. I looked for Walt. Turning my head with effort, I found him standing beside me. I searched his face. Was he anxious? Had the surgeon told him more than I knew?

"Hi. You're awake." He took my hand.

"It's gone. My breast is gone, amputated! You know that, don't you?"

"Yes, I know." He spoke too calmly, I thought. "I

consulted with the doctors, and they told me you're coming out of this in fine shape."

"It's not fine. I'll never be the same."

"But you're still alive. That's all that matters."

For a moment the bed felt awkward as I tried to return his reassuring smile. I wanted to be lifted into his arms and held close; I never liked being away from him, especially at night. And night was coming. I collapsed in fatigue. I felt his warm kiss and his firm hand.

"I'll be around. Now you need your sleep."

I sensed his quiet steps as he turned to go. He was returning to the kids now. They needed him.

Soon I became aware of nurses coming and going.

"I'm going to get you ready for the night," said one.

"We have medication for you," said another. "This will help you sleep."

The night was a restless cycle of sleeping, tossing, waking, sleeping, tossing, waking. A nurse checked in every hour on her routine rounds. The drainage pump beside my bed made a bubbling noise. Although it had been there all along, I hadn't noticed it. Now it took on strange proportions, entangling dissonant harmony and monotony into the pain I felt in my arm and shoulder. *How long? How long?*

Accustomed to darkness, I was startled by a small stream of light flowing through my window. Daylight at last! The beam was tiny, the window being obstructed by that big concrete bulkhead. From the beginning in this room, I had felt shut away from the outside world.

I began hearing footsteps in the hall. Soon someone would come; I needed a reassuring face. I was grateful when a cheery nurse entered.

"I'm going to wash your face," she said, turning up the bed. "Your breakfast tray will be up soon."

Throughout the morning routine, I felt utterly listless. I was given a bath and medication. The drainage pump was readjusted, and the house doctor came by, checking patients. How feeble my attempts to acknowledge kindness!

At last there was a lull. The last nurse left my bed turned up, a welcome relief since a comfortable position was hard to maneuver.

I yielded to wool-gathering thoughts. *I suppose I should be thanking God that I am still alive.* I tossed up a sigh. *Alive! No, I am going to die!* Premonition—I was convinced!

A surge of terror throbbed through me, bringing chills to my feet and perspiration to my forehead.

Be sensible, I told myself. *Haven't the doctors been encouraging?* My shaking hands searched for the call light. I found it, and a nurse promptly came.

"Something, Mrs. Gilseth?"

She doesn't think anything is wrong, I decided as I groped for assurance. I reached out my hand. "I think . . . something might be wrong. I . . . I . . . feel faint."

"I'll take your blood pressure," she said, reaching for the instrument. I watched her face anxiously. *Calm. yes, calm.* "You are all right, Mrs. Gilseth. Just a flash of nerves. I guess I'd better turn your bed down a bit."

I breathed a little easier. I stood back from this terror for a moment and recognized that I had felt this way before. Long ago when at home alone at the age of fourteen, I had chosen a rocking chair on the front porch where I was free to pump back and forth to quell an overwhelming fear. Strange that now this anguish, this familiar face appeared once more, just as new, just as potent. Why had I been so frightened of dying then? It was the revival tent meetings. "If you die this night, are you ready to meet your Lord?" That was the frightening question so often raised. "Dying this night—dying this night!" It took months to shake this fear. I must have given it up when nothing happened. I wanted nothing to do with the "God of the tent meeting." Now God was frowning at me again! No matter how much I wanted to pray, it would not be to him. The God of my comfort was far, far away. Insecurity wove itself tightly into the well-being I sought.

The bubbling drainage pump again gnashed at the wound in my chest. A nurse entered with medication. "Do you have much pain?" she asked, not waiting for an answer. "This will give you some relief."

"Thank you," I replied feebly. "Perhaps I will try to sleep." I wanted Walt to come. How could I be insecure with him around?

Walt came—short precious moments they were—and went. He had his work. Afterwards, I became aware, once again, of the relentless bulkhead outside my window keeping daylight away from me. I wanted people around to provide temporary relief from this morbid obsession. This obstruction was becoming a symbol of oncoming darkness.

Walt came twice a day. Once when a nurse who brought a pan of wash water was called out, I asked him to wash my face.

"You are an odd one," he said, laughing as he awkwardly wrung out the washcloth. "What are nurses paid for?" I relished the firm strength of his hands.

Although I was not prepared in my mind to see him, my pastor arrived one day. A warm, sensitive man of about fifty-five with a large, round, shiny face. He was capable of showing either grief or radiating joy. Now I was too troubled to anticipate his kindness. Instead, the "God of the tent meeting" hovered nearby. Perhaps he wanted to read Scripture; I didn't want him to do that. On the other hand, I remembered the loss of his wife and his son's loss of a hand. Life had not been easy for him lately.

"So here you are when you are so needed. We had to do all the Holy Week services without you. The choir voted to sing without your direction; they didn't want me to tell you they failed to sing all together." As he spoke he seemed to fill the whole room.

I was grateful to him. He made me feel like myself again, not the miserable wretch I had been living with for what seemed like weeks.

"Sorry about that," I said, "but I intend to be out of here soon and back again at Clearbrook." I would make no apologies. No excuses or driveling self-pity.

"You haven't seen your kids for a while, have you? Hospital rules, no kids. I saw them yesterday and thought they looked a little lost. I'm sure they will be happy to have their mom back." His rich smile brought great reassurance. *Yes, I wanted to live! I would live!*

"I hope they find clean clothes. Laundry might be their worst job."

"They're not helpless. Don't fret about that. It's good for them to take responsibility." He was almost teasing.

"I'll grant you that." I smiled at him now, acknowledging he had won.

Before he left, he handed me our church bulletin. "You must keep up with what is going on with us," he said. "Here, too, is a little book of prayers. Read them whenever you feel like it."

He was gone too soon, but he left his great spirit behind for me. I felt his presence for a long time.

Something to read? I pondered as the evening tray was taken away on that last night before I went home. I remembered a poem, "Prospice," by Robert Browning, in one of the books I brought.

> Fear death? to feel the fog in my throat,
> The mist in my face . . .

I surprised myself by daring to dwell on these words.

> I was ever a fighter, so, one fight more
> The best and the last!
> I would hate that death bandage my eyes and forbore
> And bade me creep past.
> No, let me taste the whole of it . . .

When the time came, I would take on dying with as much zest as I was taking on living. As God's child, I would be given grace to be my true self no matter what.

I closed the book. I gladly took the sleeping pill, and fell asleep. A sedative would not do for a whole night. I awoke. A stream of moonlight was shining into my room through the narrow strip at the top of the window. The bulkhead, that ominous presence, had not succeeded in keeping it out! I had not died. I was alive! Robust!

2
Going Home

I was going home! One of the hospital's "Gray Ladies" was packing my belongings into my overnight bag. She had laid out my blouse, skirt, and underthings and had untied the strings holding my hospital gown together. I would now dress myself. No bra? I no longer had a bandage; the incision would heal if it were kept dry.

Unaware of the mirror on the bathroom door, I suddenly was faced with what had happened to me. This can't be true! How ghastly! Stitches were sunk like so many black insects. A hideous blue wound filled the hollow where my left breast had been!

"See, it's not so bad, is it?" She had put down the suitcase and stood beside me, both of us looking into the mirror. She had been with me before, a motherly, nurturing type, patting my bedclothes as she smiled down on me. *How can she be honest and say such a thing?* I was angry at her. She was more naive than I expected her to be. I couldn't express my anger, however, and suddenly felt sorry for her making this attempt to comfort me.

Certainly there would be a bra—as soon as possible. And a sundress, too. As if meeting a challenge, I imagined my good shoulder and neck bare in an off-one-shoulder sundress—I would start sewing as soon as I got home. Swimsuit? That could be arranged too.

I rolled down the long antiseptic hallway in a wheelchair much to my consternation; I had hoped to walk. I came through the open door and sat dazzled! *So this is how it is outside?* The bulkhead in front of my room had hidden what little the window could have revealed. The freshness of newly-cut green grass! The rich beds of spring flowers stretched out with colors of red, yellow, pink, lavender, and white. A flowering magnolia, yes, and a burst of yellow sunlight from a forsythia shrub. The boulevard across the street was lined with flowering trees, a promenade of red. I had forgotten it was April, the State of Washington at its best. I remembered the rhododendron shrubs in our back garden. They must be blooming! And the dogwood tree in the front yard, a profusion of white would be a sentinel to greet me.

Someone helped me out of the wheelchair and into the front seat of our car that Walt had parked in the patient loading area. As we sped through traffic and onto the fifteen miles of highway toward our town, I felt as though this was the first time I had been in a car. I was in some kind of a capsule with the whole world whirling and whizzing by. *What if I were driving? No, not this time, you aren't.* I was alarmed by my sudden disorientation but reality returned when Walt spoke.

"I asked Peggy Loreen to come mornings for a week or until you feel like stirring about." He turned toward me and I caught his glance.

"She is very nice. I'll like that," I said though I hadn't counted on this.

"Steve will be home for lunch today. He's anxious to have his mom back."

In my mind's eye, I saw Steve sitting on the little red chair we'd bought for him when he began kindergarten, back when parents helped furnish the leased classroom space. Now I longed for him. I would have him back.

We stopped at the end of the sidewalk to the front door. The dogwood was just beginning to bloom. I knew it!

"Let me walk without help," I said. "I want to take my time. How beautiful everything has become!" A robin flew from a nearby shrub and onto the lawn. Louie, our old bachelor neighbor, was hoeing his garden. We always admired his row of raspberry bushes.

The house smelled of fresh furniture polish. Was this really where I lived? Not a thing out of place, even the carpet looked cleaner than I remembered it.

"Welcome home! I have a cup of tea for you whenever you're ready." Peggy was making a difference.

"Thank you, how nice."

"I must run along now," Walt looked at his watch. "But Steve will be home any minute."

Peggy and I had tea sitting on the davenport in front of the coffee table. We drank from English china cups purchased in Canada. "Nothing but the best for this occasion," explained Peggy, as if she were not sure I would approve of her using them.

"Thank you, Peggy. There is a real lift to a cup of tea," I said, and meant it.

After lunch, I again sat on the davenport with Steve by my side. He brought the book we had been reading before I left for the hospital: *The Lion, the Witch and the Wardrobe,* by C. S. Lewis.

"Hasn't anyone read to you since I've been gone? Surely . . . "

"Yes, Carolyn several times and Dad once—other books. But I saved this for you since you will want to know what happens."

"That was thoughtful of you. I do want to know what happens. So let's go to Narnia!"

"Pretty soon they'll see Aslan, the lion!" Steve found the page and settled in next to me.

Something in this story of a magic place made sense to me. The children in the tale found themselves in a strange land. Unheard of adventure awaited them. But what? Above all, there was the noble lion, Aslan:

> People who have not been in Narnia sometimes think that a thing cannot be good and terrible at the same time. If the children had ever thought so they were cured of it now. For when they tried to look at Aslan's face they just caught a glimpse of the golden mane and the great, royal, solemn, overwhelming eyes . . . his voice was deep and rich. . . . They now felt glad and quiet and it didn't seem awkward to them to stand and say nothing.

As I read, I somehow met up with Aslan, though he was a wild lion. I felt glad and quiet. The story told me he was noble and strong on behalf of those who sought his help.

After the reading we played "Peter Pan," the favorite record of the moment. Lovely thoughts will send us flying. We understood each other, Steve and I. Later when he went to join his friends, I saw my unread magazines, *The Atlantic, The Lutheran Standard,* and others piled neatly on the endtable. *Not today,* I thought, *but soon I'll get into them.*

School was out, for I heard footsteps and chatter

in the street. The door opened and in came Ron. No homework, as usual.

"Hi! Great to see you home!" he exclaimed, bouncing down the two steps into our living room.

"Hi! Great to be back. Have you been behaving yourself?"

"Come on—you know I always behave myself." Ron was outgoing and easy to tease. He turned as if in a hurry.

"Where are you going?" I asked.

"Fishing. The Nooksack is loaded with trout just now. I'll bring you some for dinner." He was gone. I heard him rattling his tackle out of the garage.

The door opened again and Carolyn came in as unhurried as Ron had been rushed and as loaded down with books as he had been empty-handed.

"Well, hi! I thought you would be here by the time I got home from school How are you? You look great!

"Thank you. That dress looks nice on you."

"Cotton dress day—remember?"

"That's right. I wouldn't have been prepared." Cotton dress day was a spring celebration—a colorful style show, really. I missed it this year.

"Wilbur Olander wants to come over. He asked if you were home. He's so shy and awkward. I'm surprised he dared talk to me. I told him you were home. Okay?"

"Fine. He's preparing for another recital, I suppose."

"S'pose so," she said, turning to leave. "Did Peggy vacuum? I have heaps of homework." She continued through the hall and up the stairs.

I glanced at the piano and remembered how it sounded that rainy night last winter when Wilbur came to play in response to my invitation. A Chopin polonaise for a special recital, he said, and he needed a preview audience. That night Wilbur pretended his visit was merely to return some magazines I had lent him. He hesitated, then left, only to return at once with a portfolio he had left in a plastic bag at the front door in the rain. It was difficult to share an area of his life as lonely as his music was. I felt honored then. Wilbur was creative. He realized a great deal from his playing and it came through for the listener. I searched for a better word than awkward, as Carolyn had expressed it—his peer's perception of him. Modesty, hanging on to a confidence in his own worth; that was better. *What now?* I wondered. I pictured him on that piano bench again. It would be a treat for me.

Peggy placed a hot dish in the oven and set the timer before she left, so I needn't worry about dinner. At least the family would be hungry. Perhaps meals at home would restore my appetite.

"Look at the trout I caught! I have two beauties—one measures all of twelve inches!" Ron came through the front door, noisy and excited.

"Let's see," I called. "Feet wet?"

He teetered on the top step, holding two rainbow trout by the tail. "I'll clean them and maybe we could fix them for dinner?"

"Sounds great," I said, not sure who would do that. I knew no one would let me into the kitchen, but perhaps someone could, with my instructions.

"What a catch!" Walt entered the kitchen with a load of groceries. "Ron's been at it again. Want them for dinner?"

"What could be better?" I replied in a lively voice. I

sighed with relief. With his enthusiasm, the fish would be prepared.

I closed my eyes only minutes before someone called, "Dinner is ready!" I carefully climbed the two steps from the living room to the dining room and sat at the table. Everyone was considerate of Mom; it gave me a nice feeling, really.

"Did it hurt much—I mean—did you feel pain when you woke up after the operation?" Ron began our table talk.

"It did. But I received a shot in my rear when I was barely awake that put me back to sleep for I don't know how long. It was late afternoon when I woke, and I thought it was still morning."

I looked at Ron. Knowing him, I appreciated his concern. He was kind; he worried about things like hurt and pain, and this was characteristically on his mind.

"This fish can't be beat, fresh out of the Nooksack," I continued, responding to Ron. "And prepared to perfection!" This was meant for Walt.

"Will you get a prosthesis?" asked Carolyn.

This would be her question. I wondered what her feeling would be on knowing what had happened to me. Would she identify and find it horrible? She was a young woman now and usually very secretive about developing breasts and menstruation. I remembered putting a bra in her dresser drawer earlier, guessing at the size, along with a box of Kotex, not knowing when she would need them.

"What's a prosthes . . . ?" blurted Steve.

"Yeah, what's that?" chimed Ron.

"An artificial part of the body. In my case, a breast." I hastened to answer for her. "I will have one when I am sufficiently healed. There's a place in Bellingham where I can be fitted. It will be worn inside my bra. I'll look great! No need for me to go around like an old hag!" *Wow—I had said quite enough!*

"You'll be going around fooling people?" Steve piped up, holding back a giggle until the rest of us laughed.

"Tomorrow night we'll have popovers. I learned to make them in Home Ec today." Carolyn changed the embarrassing subject.

We were leaving the table when the telephone rang. "It's for you," said Carolyn who had picked up the phone. "It sounds like Mr. S.," she whispered as she handed me the phone.

"Hello?"

It indeed was the co-advisor for the senior class. "As you know," he said, "graduation is only three weeks away and the committee of seniors has chosen the speakers. When will you be back? They need some coaching."

"Who are they?" I asked. "Peter Schieber will scarcely need help, just some looking over."

"We're not using Pete. He is such a ham these days, you wouldn't believe it. We're using Janice, Gary, and Don."

"I don't understand." I felt weak and sank into a chair that Walt brought for me.

"Could you stop in Monday? I know you won't be back in school yet, but I need some help with these kids."

"Yes, I'll come on Monday." I replaced the receiver slowly and looked at Walt, who I knew was ready to explode.

"What do you mean, you'll be at school on Monday? You're convalescing! You can't do that!"

"Just for an hour or so. They need me." Suddenly I felt very much alive. I had work to do. "Ron, what's the matter with Pete? Mr. S. says he is a ham."

"He's so grubby since he went to stay with that farmer. He's changed since his mother left," Carolyn began clearing the table.

"The kids still like him, but he thinks he needs to goof off," said Ron. "He's really not himself when he does that. Remember how good he was in the class play? And the time he did that part out of Shakespeare you liked so well—that the kids thought was so corny? And he's a violin player—who cares about that? He did kick for the football team; that won the kids. Doesn't Mr. S. want him to be a class speaker at graduation?"

"That's the problem." I wanted Ron to continue.

"Mr. S. doesn't like Pete. He's too smart for him. Pete knows more than the teacher, and that's a fact."

"Maybe he can help the others write their speeches," put in Carolyn, who listened as she stacked dishes.

"Not too bad an idea. The kids respect him for all he knows," continued Ron.

"Maybe we can have him play his violin." I tried this out on them.

"That would be cool!" Ron was satisfied.

There was something about Pete that made it easy to disregard him. He was far from being dashing and frequently made a nuisance of himself. He hadn't learned the proper restraints that an average teacher looks for in better students. I knew why Pete wasn't speaking, and I resented Mr. S. and the whole group who refused to accept him.

Walt carried in a log for the fireplace. "A bit chilly

toward evening," he said. Each of the others returned to their own concerns and we were left alone.

"The doorbell—who could that be?" Walt, with a good fire going, went to the door.

It was Wilbur. Even before he entered, I saw his plastic sack of music.

"Come in, Wilbur. You're here to see Mrs. Gilseth? She's right here." Walt was congenial enough.

I invited him in, and he sat on the piano bench. Yes, his recital was coming up and he was to play another Chopin piece, a nocturne this time. He especially liked Chopin, he said. I understood. They were perhaps alike and would have been kindred spirits.

A light came into his eyes when I encouraged him to play. It was a treat for me as I knew it would be. He had carefully memorized his selection with attention to interpretation out of his gifted imagination. When he finished, he picked up his plastic sack, quickly said goodnight, and was gone.

"So? You're back in the swing of things," said Walt coming out of the study. "I'll bet you're tired."

"Not really, but I'll let you put me to bed. I'm spoiled with all that attention the nurses gave me."

"I knew it!" he said, laughing.

I was home!

3
Facing Old Friends

As I climbed the stairs with Walt's supporting arm around me, I was overcome by a sudden realization. This was not one of those nurses or hospital orderlies or just anyone being helpful and kind. No, this was my lover. We were going to our bedroom and would lie side by side again. No more cranking up the bed or raising guardrails. No more bedpans and sleeping pills would be necessary. Now I would give way to a sweet reassurance of well-being.

"Peggy made up our bed—fresh for us." He sat me on a chair. "Here, let me take off your shoes."

"I can manage the rest," I said, feeling his hand squeezing each of my feet. "On second thought, I could let you undress me."

Off went skirt, blouse, and underthings—but no bra to unhook. How matter-of-fact he was as he went about hanging up each garment. Didn't he see for himself what had happened to me?

"I'll go downstairs for a pitcher of water and a glass—you got used to that, didn't you? And maybe another blanket. I'll see about it."

After he left the room, I went to the mirror and dared to look at myself. No, how could he love me anymore! Even when this healed there would be a horrid scar! No prosthesis would do when it came right down to being me—whole, acceptable me—who was his wife! Mutilation! Something profoundly evil had happened to me. I felt medieval, a repulsive creature of those days, a witch! Hearing his foot hit the top step, I pulled on my nightgown.

"What's the matter? You're not crying, are you?" He paused before setting down the water pitcher.

"I don't know—I guess I'm just tired." I felt myself trembling.

"We'll get you under the blankets," he said, pulling back the spread and lifting the covers. "I think you got a chill."

He propped my pillow and helped me in. "I'll be with you in a minute to warm you up." I hid my face in the pillow and let the tears come. Then I felt his warm arms reaching my way.

"I'm never going to be the way I used to be," I began. "I don't expect you to feel about me the way you used to," I struggled to continue. "I've lost such a vital part of myself . . . I mean love-making can never be the same."

"Are you crazy? I have my lover back! I'm so fortunate. You know I might have lost you! One lovely breast is as good as two. Come now, I want to hold you, warm you up. I've missed you. You've been gone many nights, you know." He caught me and held me close to him. "Oops, I can't be reckless until you heal."

I wasn't sure sleeping-in was a luxury that morning as the bedrooms emptied and I was left alone. By the time I came downstairs, Peggy had already cleared away the breakfast dishes and set my place at the table.

"It's quiet and peaceful again," Peggy began as she

brought a cup of coffee and seated herself across from me. "You must try these cinnamon rolls Evelyn Howell brought this morning." She passed the plate to me. "You do live on a neighborly street."

Did these women bringing food feel sorry for me, pity me? I wondered. *Are they whispering among themselves about what had happened to me?* I felt a fleeting resentment. No. Acts of kindness should be taken at face value.

"I think I'll visit the back yard for a while," I told Peggy when we finished our breakfast.

"Take a sweater, then. It's a bit cool," she called after me.

Our little brown terrier was on her feet ready to follow me out. Her name was Brownie, but she was seldom called just that. Most often she was "Brown Dog" or "Brown Hound" or what any one of us cared to call her. She was old now. We took her from the dog pound in Seattle when our foster children first came to us at ages five and eight. She was really a house dog and never left the yard. When Ron was younger, Brownie shared his bedroom in the basement. We used to say she understood the Lord's Prayer because it was a signal for her to lead the way to bed following the family's evening devotion. When Steve was a baby, Brownie took over guarding the baby carriage if I chanced to leave it a minute or two. She snoozed on a pillow in our study while we corrected papers and prepared our lessons. She was so settled into our routine that she was easy to ignore, but some day we were really going to miss her.

She was an old dog now. The vet told us our little friend had diabetes—we fed her too much sugar—let her lick the frosting bowl—and we shouldn't have. She was losing weight. She used to be fat, now she was about the right size, but there was an ashen look about her eyes that troubled me. Her coat lacked luster. Put her to sleep? No, we all agreed, not yet. I had a troubling kinship with her as I looked into her eyes and reached out to pet her. Not yet—but soon?

"So here you are already enjoying this beautiful day." Clara Anderson came through the backdoor, looking for me. "Peggy said I would find you here. My, you look as fresh and wholesome as the flowers!"

Clara and her husband Elmer were friends from Clearbrook Church, a rural Lutheran congregation of the then Swedish Augustana Synod. At first we wondered whether driving seven miles out in the country to go to church was feasible since there were other churches, both Methodist and Presbyterian, in town. After our first worship, our whole family was convinced that it was.

At that time we had moved from metropolitan Seattle, where we were members of a large church with not much chance to get acquainted. Steve had been unwilling to stay in the preschool Sunday school class there, but at Clearbrook, to my astonishment, he took Clara's hand and readily went off with her. "We are friends of Jesus," she said.

"I'm doing great, thanks to all the tender, loving care I'm getting," I said, responding to her warm embrace. "Find a place to sit. How's Elmer? Busy with fieldwork, I imagine."

"Oh, yes, always busy on the farm. He sends his love."

How Elmer captivated us all, I'll never know. No one escaped his magnetism. He attracted teenagers, encouraging them to organize game nights in the church annex, an old school gym with basketball hoops at each end. This was great for Ron who, in Seattle, was scared to go to school for fear of a neighborhood bully who he said was after him. Carolyn also found friends her age in this gathering of cheerful people.

"Tell him I can't wait to hear his next story. What's new?"

"The choir sang again without you—twice now—but we can't get by much longer." A sudden smile. "Last Sunday Elmer got a kick out of one of the altos. As she left her pew to go with the choir to sing, her foot caught in the handle of someone's purse and she dragged it into the aisle before she got free of it." Clara laughed heartily as she always did at Elmer's humor.

I laughed too, recalling that wonderful group of people who supported me even now. The embarrassing purse incident was a laughable anecdote that would remain around for a long time. This magical man made everyone feel good; burdens were lifted by such a simple thing as a laugh.

Peggy joined us, bringing a pot of coffee and a plate of nut bread. She, too, was a member of Clearbrook Church. "You can't imagine what Clara brought you! Your whole dinner: ham, potato salad, baked beans, and chocolate cake with fudge frosting! Won't you love it!"

"Yes. I can imagine it, knowing Clara." I said, struck again by this woman's generosity toward others and gaining such joy from it.

Pastor M., another visitor from Clearbrook Church, also came that afternoon. Remembering the reassurance I received during his hospital visit, I welcomed him with warm affection. He sat in an armchair across from me so we could have eye contact. A stream of sunshine from the southwest entered through a window.

"It's easy to see that you're recovering well," he began with a ready smile.

"It s good to be out of the hospital and home again," I responded. As we visited I recalled giving him one of my short stories to read not long ago. It might serve as a frame of reference for the topic we both were eager to reach. "Have you found time to read my short story?" I asked. My question seemed like an abrupt change of subject.

He leaned forward, "Yes, indeed. I read it with great interest, and I'm glad you brought it up. I've wondered how much of what you related in this story would disturb you these days?"

"The Eucharist" is a short sketch of a woman suffering from postnatal anxiety tension, modeling my own experience following the premature birth and death of our second son. At that time I fell into a pit of a dread I was unable to escape for more than a year. Depression or melancholy were useless words to describe the unreal, irrational fear that overwhelmed me.

"No, none of that horrible unreality has clutched me now. I feel insecure, perhaps, but nothing I'm not able to handle. Dr. Brown told me that since I lived through those fears once, I would not be as vulnerable again. Now I believe him."

"That is wonderful." He paused as if I had more to say.

"I did experience a flash of that death dread described in the story, but only for a moment," I added.

"You sound quite confident. May I ask now how you

lived through your fear, as your doctor called it?" asked Pastor M.

"That's partly answered by the experience in 'The Eucharist,' the point of the story. Of course, there is the matter of faith—belief in the love of God that will not let us go, come what may."

"That sounds like a pious cliché," he said, challenging me.

"Not if one has sincerely experienced it. Surely you've read more of Kierkegaard than I have, but there I found insights into the mystery of God's love. One quote I remember is:

> He [God] gives to pain a significance which almost overwhelms me. . . . Our security does not lie in being like others, but in single-minded trust in the God of love.

"No, I am not always confident. But I know where true confidence may be found."

"What can I say? You've said it all!" He sat back in his chair and folded his hands across his chest.

"By no means have I said it all."

I felt humble before this man who had so recently lost his wife. He was living out his faith for all of us to see. Clearbrook was his parish, and we all drew strength from him.

"Thanks for letting me read your story. Psychology is an interest of mine. More people than we know are filled with silent terror and need the healing touch of God's love." After a reflective pause, he continued, "I wish you luck sending your story out. It has a vital message." *Sending it out? Might it be published? Should I pursue it?*

As he rose to go, he said, "I look forward to having you back at worship. It is an inspiration seeing you in the pew." He had given me much this day, and I hoped he would find time to return.

Pastor M. left just as the children returned from school. Among the usual crowd was an unexpected drop-in, Peter Schieber, the senior who had been denied the right to speak at commencement. I chose a corner of the backyard where we could talk with the privacy I knew he needed.

"I'm so glad you're back. I've thought about you a lot and wished you well even if you didn't get a card from me." He sprawled on a bench at the picnic table with his feet out in front of him. "I didn't want to be just another name on your cards. That's too easy."

"How do you mean that—just another name?" I was comfortable in a lawn chair opposite him.

"I guess I needed to see you to tell you. No way could I get to the hospital. Otherwise I would've."

"Thank you, Peter. I appreciate your friendship and concern; believe me." To prevent an awkward pause I continued. "What's new?"

He sat up straight. "I got the scholarship from Reed. We made it!"

"What do you mean, we?"

"The essay on liberal education. You helped me—remember?"

Yes, I remembered the urgency he felt. I had been an audience, merely a supportive listener because the essay had real merit, masterfully done. "Great news! I must say I thought it a very impressive piece of work, so I'm not really surprised. Now you're on your way. You are to be congratulated."

"Thanks." He pulled his feet back under the bench and looked away for a moment.

Was he grubby the way Carolyn described him? His plaid shirt was grimy and limp, his faded jeans were worn thin at the knees. His hair was too long. I resolved then and there to call his house mother at the place he stayed to be sure he had a proper shirt to wear at graduation. I would do something about a haircut, too. I wasn't about to hear comments about grubbiness that evening.

Peter looked at me with serious eyes. He had not changed so far as I could see. His broad shoulders had strength still, and his integrity was apparent. "I'm not speaking at graduation although you perhaps thought I would."

"I've heard. Mr. S. called me."

"I hoped I might. I had some good ideas you would have liked."

"I'm sure of that. How much does it matter to you?" Surely he must be hurting, and I didn't seem to be of much help.

"Well, I've only been with the class two years. I guess I shouldn't have expected it." He looked into the trees as though he had found a satisfactory answer.

I looked at this young man who had just received a scholarship at a prestigious college for having written an essay on liberal education, but who was grievously disregarded by the administration and faculty of his high school. I was baffled.

"Why don't you share your ideas with Janice?" I asked. "She would catch on and run with them."

"I already have. Gary and Don have asked me for help, too."

"Okay, right on! Ghost writer, another of your

roles!" He laughed with me. "I'm still anxious to see the poem you told me you were writing," I said, changing the subject.

Peter stuck his hand in the back pocket of his jeans and pulled out a square of folded yellow paper. He took time to unfold it and smooth the creases before handing it to me. "It's rather abstract, as you say much of what I write turns out to be. I tried to incorporate images as you suggested once."

"You read it," I coaxed.

"No, you. I want to hear it read to me by another person. I'll pretend I'm hearing it for the first time."

The poem was titled "Distance." What did he mean? Space, room for movement, life and being. Philosophy? Indeed. Space!

> "Distance
> Thou must span great and small, and so unerring
> venture forth to span this world . . . and beyond it, all."

I read, without stopping, the three twelve-line stanzas. At the end my voice lowered and my hands fell into my lap.

"What do you think?" he asked.

"I'm challenged. I know once I absorb all you have included here, I'm going to like it. Infinity, what a scope you have chosen. Let me read the opening line to each verse once more:

> "Distance of East, distance of North, be . . .
> Distance of South, distance of West, fall . . .
> Distance of Knowing, distance of Love, endure.

"And in between are all the images."

Peter simply looked at me rather than defining what he meant. I liked that about him.

"Will you let me keep this for a while?" I asked.

"That copy is for you."

Our visit ended and as I watched him cut across the lawn and onto the road, I realized how lonely he was. Perhaps he always would be, but he would continue to like people for whatever response they gave him. I identified with that. My surgery had been an experience that could not be readily shared, so I would now have to compensate. No matter. I now had a new kind of energy to use for however long I lived—searching, writing, teaching, listening. No matter how many days I had, none could be wasted. *Today is now,* I thought, *and must be lived to the fullest.*

Since Walt had an early evening meeting, I settled before the fireplace to read Peter's poem over several times. I sat back and felt a new dimension in my environment. The last stanza read:

> Distance of Knowing, distance of Love,
> Endure. Frost not thy pane with age,
> Silent . . . conduct a life above
> The meagerness of speaking things. Be stage
> To character and human form;
> Be motherly . . . direct but wise;
> Stand resolute throughout the storm
> Of human truths and human lies.
> Be not a wall, unmoved to change
> Or circumstance, but only space
> Reflecting bolder images at range
> And leaving time its own great destiny to trace.

4

Summer 1957, Living with a Prosthesis

I was prepped in a white hospital gown, told to sit in a high leather chair and wait. "He'll be right in," said the nurse.

Ten minutes passed, but I understood the delay. Dr. B.'s patients always waited a long time since he never rushed anyone. "Have the stitches begun to bother you? When they feel uncomfortable, they need to come out." Dr. B. arrived at last. "You're looking good—healing well," he said. "We'll try not to hurt you." He smiled as the nurse brought the tray of snippers and tweezers. The twisted threads were slowly drawn out—nothing traumatic about it—just one by one, until the last.

I resented those stitches sewn in my chest wall. Something was gone and the empty space sealed forever. Now, since my body decided I could get along without that part of me, the stitches were taken away. Dr. B. told me to wait a month before being fitted for a breast prosthesis and handed me a brochure advertising that service. "And that's it," he said. "You needn't come back unless you have a problem."

I was discharged. What needed to be done had been done.

The next month I entered the largest pharmacy in Bellingham hoping to find the orthopedic appliance department. Showing my brochure as a pass, I was led to a corner at the back of the store where canes, wheelchairs, and various obscure contraptions were kept. I was greeted by a mature woman who smiled and said, "Come right in here." We walked through a curtained door to a small fitting room with a large mirror. "Have you waited long enough for all swelling to go down?"

"I've been wearing a bra for more than a week now, and I'm using a makeshift pad for the time being."

"You evidently sew," she said, noticing how I had improvised my enhancer. "That will help since you need to sew pockets in your bras for your prothesis." This woman reminded me of the Gray Lady at the hospital, although she was far more sophisticated and sensitized to her job.

She found the name brand Identical Form, size six, among a pile of boxes on a shelf in the storeroom and brought it to me, holding it gently. Obviously, I wasn't merely trying on a pair of shoes.

"I think you already realize that your prosthesis must have the same weight as your other side for the sake of your back." She gave it to me to examine, then went back to the storeroom and brought out a bra with a pocket.

What a preposterous contraption, I thought. *No thanks. Not for me!* She must have sensed my dissatisfaction for she whisked it away and brought an envelope with an enclosed pattern. "If you wish to make your own pockets, here is what you want."

Being new at this, I accepted it, although I still thought it quite preposterous as I looked it over and tried to imagine how I would use it. She closed the lid on the box, handed it to me, and said, "Now watch out. Don't get reckless and stick a pin in it. Be careful of people who pin corsages!"

I thanked her and left, after paying the bill of $12.50. (Years later I learned this was really a bargain compared to what I subsequently had to pay for a prosthesis—$100 and finally $250.)

I did find great comfort in my recent purchase as I began using it. It was made of a soft plastic, the side toward the body made of foam. It came with two nylon mittens, easy to remove and launder. Not bad. Ignoring the clerk's instructions about sewing pockets, I simply placed my "Identical Form" into my bra and wore it. Its weight was perfect; no doubt that was the reason no other form would do.

Our clothesline, only a few steps from the basement door, ran parallel to our boundary hedge. The spacious lawn was kept free for lounging, outdoor eating, and play. This beautiful June morning I brought out a basket of laundry—too nice a day to waste on the dryer. Summer vacation had begun. I was free of school responsibilities, and it felt good to resume my normal activities as I felt able, following the instructions of my doctor. I decided that hanging out the wash was good exercise for me since I had been told to raise my left arm often to improve its flexibility. I was impressed with how easy it was to reach the lines and pinch the pins. At this point I often forgot, for days at a time, that I was wearing a prosthesis, or that I ever had surgery. It was others, who had not caught up with me, that reminded me of my misfortune.

I thought about summer and all its possibilities.

The garden looked fine; there would be tomatoes to can and beans to freeze. The raspberry bushes, pruned last fall, would yield an abundance. I saw two apple trees with prospects of a good harvest, the blossoms had been so prolific. I would like a "getaway" trip somewhere, maybe east of the Cascade Mountains, warmer than here—a place to camp, swim with the kids, and lie in the sun. Perhaps Sun Lakes Park where Walt and Ron could play golf.

Early summer also meant sewing—turning out cotton dresses and shorts for the coming season. I returned my basket to the basement, commending my wash to the fragrant fresh air, and decided to go shopping for fabrics. I would make that off-the-shoulder playsuit I had resolved to do while still in the hospital. There was nothing to stop me from showing off my beautiful shoulders!

I browsed through pattern books at Lynden Department Store and found what I was looking for. Then I searched for bolts of fabric in the crowded aisles. Polka dots—that would be it—red, orange, yellow, and black on an off-white background. I brought the bolt and the pattern to the cashier.

"So your daughter will have a new summer outfit," said Linda, assessing the pattern. "Lucky girl she is!"

"If you say so," I replied with a smile. She needn't know that Carolyn bought her own material and sewed her own clothes, or that this outlandish pattern and polka dot material were for me. I realized I was being too sensitive and resentful toward people these days. Linda was good-hearted and pleasant.

"I would like to take a look at your swimwear," I said, turning toward the women's department.

"Some new ones came in a week ago." Linda followed me.

"No plunging neckline, please," I said to let her know it was for me and that I intended to swim like all the rest of humanity this season.

"We'll take a look," she said and smiled.

But when we came to the circular rack of women's swimwear, I grew apprehensive. They seemed to be so much nothing, the shoulder straps merely strings. And I certainly didn't want yellow—black, maybe.

"How about this—slightly built-up shoulders, a plunging back, and a little sham skirt?" She pulled out two suits of the same style, one black, the other blue with white figures.

"That's pretty close," I replied. I assessed the built-up strap and decided I could sew in a pocket with a zipper enclosure. Ingenious!

"Just right?" Linda must have caught my approval. She beamed.

"I'll take the blue one," I replied, checking the size. After buying two zippers—one a four-inch and the other a nine-inch—and matching sewing thread for my two projects, I returned home.

There I found a letter from my sister Ruth in Minot, North Dakota. I dropped my parcels on the couch, sat down, and read the letter that mentioned plans for getting together that summer. "It's been such a long time since we have seen each other; this must be a family reunion," she wrote. "We've been so busy working and raising our families that we have neglected each other."

I looked up for a moment. *Does she think I'm going to die? We can't put this off any longer?*

Ruth suggested that all of us attend Mount Carmel

Bible Camp at Medicine Lake for a week. No meals to fix; lots of time to visit. Sister Helen could come from Minneapolis with her family and possibly our brother Carl and his wife, Valborg. There would be adequate accommodations, lots of play area for kids, including a safe swimming beach—what could be nicer! "This year," she continued, "an excellent musician is scheduled to be there—we could do some singing. What do you say? Would the week of July 15th work out for you?"

I hadn't been back to Minnesota, my home state, for several years. It would be good to be there again during summer. Steve could get acquainted with his cousins. Ron would stay behind since he had a farm job with the Andersons. Carolyn could choose to pick beans or go with us—perhaps she would have had enough of field work after the strawberry season finished. Walt would be willing; he had mentioned a possible trip east earlier. The idea began to sound exciting. I would have a place to wear my sundress, and to swim. I was prepared to show my sisters that I was not in the least disturbed by what had happened to me.

Though not related either to family or directly to our Bible camp activities at Mount Carmel, events occurred that would radically change the course of our lives. We met Leigh and Helen Johnson who, in a matter of months, would be on their way to Africa to work in a teacher-training college on the mission field of the Augustana Lutheran Church in Tanganyika (later Tanzania), East Africa. The need for teachers, they said, had grown in the last few years. Their daughter Martha, three years old, would go with them, eventually attending a school for American children on the field. Leigh would teach courses in English to African students, who had completed eight to ten years of school to become elementary teachers in their country. As a matter of course, Leigh and Helen would learn Swahili, the country's language, in order to fit into the local African church community. Helen, a nurse, would work at the area's busy clinic where competent personnel were in short supply.

Following the conversation with them, Walt opened the subject again that evening as we lingered under the stars before bedtime. "What do you think about what Leigh and Helen are doing?"

"Absolutely great!" I said. "I wish we could do something like that. Being settled like we are doesn't strike me as rewarding any more—not that I don't appreciate our good jobs. But we seem to be in a rut. I see others around me in a rut, neighbors, colleagues. I don't think this is all there is." I sat down on the cabin steps to delay going indoors.

"You mean living in the best part of town in a house we were overjoyed to buy?" he teased. "Seriously, I agree with you." He sat down beside me.

"Being in a rut means isolation from so much out there—being petty about trivia in our close-knit groups. I especially feel it now. The best years of our lives must be considered."

"I talked with Leigh a lot today. He and Helen just finished a year at the seminary in Maywood, Illinois, taking mission courses, a requirement the board makes. It was a profitable time for him, he said, because he was able to take education courses at a nearby university in preparation for work as a teacher."

"How about that?" I broke in. "You could get going on a master's!"

"Wait a minute! You sound like we've already decided to take off!"

"We can dream, can't we?"

"You're really serious about this, aren't you?" What Walt was saying frightened me a bit.

"It's a big decision, I grant you." I noticed my voice changing.

"Leigh gave me the address and phone number of their headquarters. They could send particulars."

"So you've gone that far. You're serious, too, then."

"We have a year to think it over." He rose and opened the cabin screen door.

After a swim the following afternoon, Ruth, Helen, and I sat on the beach, poking our feet in the warm sand. The kids were in the water with Carolyn—bless her—watching them. She decided not to pick beans and came with us. I hoped she was having a good time even though she was older than the rest of our brood and shy about getting acquainted with other campers her age. Just now she was having a water fight with Clinton, age ten.

"Howard tells me Walt and Leigh Johnson have had serious talks about Africa. What's going on?" Ruth began as she piled sand over her ankles.

"Both of us, being teachers, might do some good there." I sounded as casual as possible.

"Really! You're thinking about it?" Ruth's voice sounded incredulous.

"Nothing's decided, but yes, we're thinking about it."

"Being missionaries?" Helen, who had been leaning on her elbows, sat up straight.

"I don't see us under a tree with savages, if that's

what you're thinking." I laughed and waited for them to laugh. "We'd be teachers in a classroom teaching English."

"Do you feel called? Maybe this is just fascination with a novel idea," Helen continued.

"Seriously, that is a good question." I paused to gather my thoughts. "Recognizing need and . . . having a desire to act . . . could that not be call, as you say?" They both nodded lamely. "From early childhood we've learned about overseas mission work. We were taught to value that work and were fascinated by stories of those who returned on furlough. I think this has a subconscious grip on us, however vague. Becoming a missionary could have been up there with becoming a fireman or a nurse."

"But what if you need medical attention?" Ruth was asking.

I knew this was coming. I felt their eyes on the contoured bustline of my new swimsuit.

"It's not like the old days. There are doctors and I can return home by plane in a matter of days." I hadn't thought of that. *Am I handicapped now?* I hadn't faced the possibility before. "I'll just have to take my chances with the rest." I tried to keep from sounding annoyed.

"Four years is a long time. It's as long as since we last saw each other—long time, no see," Helen put in. I hadn't expected enthusiasm in this matter, but when I needed something from my family, they were there for me.

Shortly after returning home, we drove to Anderson's to retrieve our little Brown Dog who came running out to meet us. We stood open-mouthed, for she was literally a skeleton! Her diabetes had progressed to the point where food no longer nourished her. "Sorry, but that's the way it is," said Ron, seeing our astonishment.

Brown Dog happily jumped into the car, knowing she was on her way home. Her eyes that greeted us with so much love were large and unnatural in their sockets. The coat we remembered as sleek, was an unhealthy gray.

"She eats her food and seems happy enough," Clara said, trying to soften the blow for us. "But one can see she's not well."

"She is twelve years old . . . that's eighty-four years of dog life," said Ron.

We drove home in silence. No doubt Ron had a lot to talk about, but that would have to wait. Reaching home, we lingered in the car. "We must take her right away," I said firmly.

"If she is still peppy, as Clara said, why not let her live a little longer?" Walt and Ron both agreed. We got out of the car, leaving it in the driveway.

"She's suffering—starving to death!" Carolyn said.

"I'll take her right now! Anyone want to go with me?" My resolve hit home. I gathered my little friend in my arms and looked into the faces of my family. Would anyone come? I guess not. I drove along Front Street, my little friend beside me. Just she and I. She soon to die—soon to die! The time had come to die!

There was no doubt in the face of our vet as to what I wanted when I handed over the emaciated little creature. I looked into her trusting eyes. "Thanks for everything," I whispered. "Good-bye."

"You don't want the carcass, do you? I have to ask." He spoke so softly that I hardly heard, but I understood.

"No," I said.

On the way home, I thought of how soon this moment had come—unexpectedly soon. That's the way it is, always unexpectedly soon! My time, unexpectedly soon!

Christmas was near. I was sewing. I tried on an unfinished blouse and stood before the mirror in our bedroom. As I drew one arm into the sleeve, I noticed a tiny rise in the scar alongside of my bra strap. It was small, like a grain of sand, nothing! Or was it? Recurrence was my dread—the possibility of it—my terror! I stripped down and rechecked. I felt and felt! *No, scars are uneven and bumpy. You are exaggerating. You are out of control. Calm down!*

I managed to let it pass—for now.

5

September 1958, Planning for Tanganyika

I sat shivering on a sheet-covered table in the clinic examining room, clad only in a hospital gown tied in the back, waiting for the doctor. Would I be qualified for the Tanganyika assignment? Would I be labeled a risk? Or worse, would the grain of sand near the scar be diagnosed as a recurring malignancy?

Until now our plans had gone well; a step at a time had led us to this moment. Following our interview, the mission board's executive director responded positively to our request. After completing our final year of teaching in Washington State, we put our house up for sale and found renters for the interim. We sold all our furniture except for the piano, which we shipped to my brother's house in Minneapolis, Minnesota.

Ron and Carolyn were left behind in Washington. Ron joined the navy on finishing high school, and Carolyn was granted permission by her case worker to stay with a family in Lynden to finish her final year of high school. After ten years I hadn't come to terms with parting with the two of them, nor would I ever—the anguish of foster parenting is another story.

My brother—and Walt's sister—Carl and Valborg Chrislock, at whose home in Minneapolis we now stayed, were shocked at the direction our lives were taking. But something had happened in me that loomed too large for explanation. It was vaguely expressed in Peter's poem: "Distance of knowing, distance of loving . . . frost not thy pane . . . " *There must be something more before life is over,* I thought, and Walt's feelings were akin to mine. After working as an insurance agent, he had finished education courses and chosen teaching as his second career—this venture was an exciting opportunity.

Knocking, but not waiting for a response, the doctor entered the examining room and took my hand in greeting, the usual "bedside" manner of most physicians. "You're a healthy woman as far as your test results show," he began as he perched a pair of glasses on his nose and stared at the clipboard he held. He looked small inside his crisp white jacket, not young, but mature enough to be flexible.

"I guess I haven't been anything but," I responded as he listened, poked, and took my blood pressure.

"No blood pressure problems," he said, replacing the contraption in its hook on the wall. I held my breath as he probed the scar on my left chest wall. "A nice job of surgery here." He reached the vulnerable spot. "A protruding bit of scar in a stitch right here." He pushed up his glasses as he looked at me. "Nothing, I would say. You might keep an eye on it—you know where I mean?"

"Yes." I gave no inkling of how relieved I was.

There were no further hurdles. We were accepted by the Augustana Mission Board to teach at Marangu Teacher Training College at seven thousand feet up the side of Mount Kilimanjaro in Tanganyika, East Africa. We were overjoyed! We had a short orientation at a missionary conference that same week where we met people who were serving in the area where we were bound, as well as families like ourselves who were on their way. One family bound for Tanganyika would spend the coming school year with us at Lutheran School of Theology, Maywood, Illinois, taking mission courses.

"You mean you're taking courses for credit?" Jean asked incredulously. (She and her husband were going to Japan.) We were folding clothes as they came out of the dryers in the basement of our seminary living quarters. We women had our role wherever we found ourselves.

"This is a chance of a lifetime for me. I've always been interested in theology, but until now I wondered why a woman should be so inclined." I tossed another batch of dry laundry on the table. "The mission courses sound interesting, especially those on world religions and history—Buddhism, wouldn't that interest you? I know I will like the biblical study in Mark, and may find others. I have the time. My boy is in second grade and gone all day."

"I will certainly audit whenever I can," she said, sounding as though she wanted this to be the end of it.

I was waving my new-found silver lining around and perhaps had just now threatened someone. I didn't tell her I had interviewed for a master's degree and was granted permission to take a non-mission course, History of Christian Thought. None of this included language study, which was left until we entered our respective countries, or what we could pick up in books, such as *Teach Yourself Swahili.*

If courses were not always accepted with enthusiasm, the fellowship we ten or so families had in this mission apartment house was akin to group therapy in that we shared the anxieties and expectations we had in common. Besides nightly devotions we scheduled potlucks, first aid classes, and discussion sessions dealing with anticipated problems of all sorts. We had no idea of precisely what each would be coping with. For example, how could Bill know that he would haul water to his living quarters from a hole several miles away, and that he couldn't escape bringing the frogs and tadpoles that came along in his barrel. Or that his latrine was so far from the house that no one went there after dark for fear of leopards. Or that we would need to seal all our food in tins to protect it from invading rats. Or that we would attack bats with tennis rackets in our house at bedtime. Risk-takers we were, but not without apprehension.

I turned forty during this time. Walt and Steve observed it with me along with the usual birthday serenade. Walt bought a little cake at the bakery and covered it with four candles, one for each decade. Steve gave me his gift: measuring spoons and salt-and-pepper shakers from Woolworth's. "You'll need them when we get to Africa," he announced. (Indeed we were in the process of gathering practical take-alongs.)

Life begins at forty!! What was wonderful about being forty? There was a freedom at this age that I had not experienced before. And now conscious that my days had become more precious, I could be more objective. I could listen to ideas, learn to know people from situation to situation without being self-conscious. I was sure I had fewer prejudices. I might not be as wildly passionate, but my appreciation of life had deepened by years of new insights. I was completely open to my remaining years! Yet I was not entirely free from my childhood phobia, namely, fear of imminent death.

"Let's skip the part where Jesus dies on the cross," said Steve one evening as we read Bible stories at bedtime.

"What then?" *Is this the same sort of dread I have?*

"Here He is alive again, walking with two guys on the road." He turned the page and showed me a picture.

I was anxious a few nights later when we came upon the story of the stoning of Stephen. Would he identify—his name and all?

And Stephen fell asleep; he awoke in heaven, I read, and looked at him.

"Is dying like falling asleep?" he asked.

"I believe it is—like in the story—don't you?"

"Then it's not very scary." I detected a tinge of bravado.

"Christians have already begun living everlasting life," I ventured, "So we are—"

"Have I begun living everlasting life?"

"Yes, indeed. It began when you were baptized."

His wriggling down under the blankets, determining an end of the session, triggered comfort. With him, this questioning and answering had taken on a refreshing newness. I was again hearing these threadbare truths as if for the first time. I kissed him on the forehead and turned out the light.

Walking out of the room, I suddenly shuddered. Would he soon see his mother "falling asleep?" *He mustn't! He needs his mother, he is only a little boy!* But would he?

The familiar fear was back, always finding new inroads, but the same dreaded emotion. I went to bed.

I fought it many hours. I wasn't coping. What a beautiful word in our vocabulary these days, coping! I wasn't and I knew it. *From whence cometh my help? My help cometh from the Lord who made heaven and earth.* I was hearing echoes. Of course, I knew *from whence* . . . I tossed and turned, trembling. *Fear and trembling,* yes, my old friend Soren Kierkegaard. He had been of help before. Value fear and trembling, it's the important prelude to faith. Faith is absurd (one of his useful words); it attaches to what cannot be grasped or understood: it's a leap. Coping right now was not the answer. It was no use seeking the answer by looking inward. In fear and trembling, leap! Let go! Let God! I finally slept.

Coping was not a bad word on the mundane level. I decided to invite Gracie over to check the grain in my scar, a prudent bid for reassurance. Both she and her husband were doctors on their way to India. In our apartment after class, she looked at our half-filled barrels—we would eventually fill fourteen of them—and exclaimed, "It looks like something is definitely going on here. And you're still sewing." She glanced toward the open machine strewn with colorful print pieces. "I wish I could sew."

"You have sewn stitches I would never dare to sew." I laughed as I found a place for us to sit. I undressed to the waist.

"What a nice job of surgery," she began like all the rest.

"I've been told that," I said.

"No kidding. You had a skilled surgeon."

"I believe you."

Gracie had found the right spot. "Here, you mean?"

"Yes."

"I honestly don't think you should let this worry you." She continued to feel around it. "Of course, if it starts to enlarge or change, you might have it looked at again. But for now, since your blood test is normal . . . and you have a clean lung x-ray . . . I wouldn't worry." She gave me a reassuring smile.

"I believe you," I said gratefully.

Someone knocked at the kitchen door. "See who it is while I get myself dressed."

It was Bill, our Canadian friend, once a prisoner of war. Bill, a German who was captured by the British and was now a citizen of Canada, would be serving with us in Tanganyika. He was loaded down with what might be the makings of our dinner.

"I want to try out my new pressure cooker, but I don't dare to do it by myself for fear it will blow up." He put his parcels on the table and the cooker on the nearest burner of the stove.

"You expect meat in Africa to be tough?" Gracie commented as she saw him unwrap a chunk of pot roast.

"I was talked into buying it. Out where I'm going, you can't get along without it, someone said. Fast, safe, and sanitary—I don't know about the safe part." By now he had covered the table with his makings. "Aren't you taking one to India?" He stopped and looked at Gracie.

"We haven't bought one yet. Should we?"

"Not because I say so," he said as he folded away a grocery sack. "It all waits to be seen." (This was to be the only time Bill ever used his pressure cooker. When in Naburara he had an African cook and didn't dare to suggest he use it.)

Gracie picked up her books. “I have to go now. Have a good meal and we'll see you at devotions. And . . . don't forget tomorrow we all line up for our first shots. I'll be waiting for you.” She nudged Bill and gave me a wink as she escaped out the door.

As for shots, all of us suffered from our first cholera inoculation and Steve spent a day in bed following his diphtheria booster. Since he was the oldest child of our group, it became his duty to be the brave one and set an example for the younger ones to follow. Gracie saw to that, and he measured up admirably.

There was a knock on the door. “Are you the folks who ordered a washing machine?” A uniformed hauler shoved a huge carton into the kitchen. “It's ready for overseas shipping,” he announced as he handed Walt the clipboard for his signature. Things were happening in earnest.

“I don't suppose my bike will fit into a barrel.” Steve came from his bedroom with an armload of books. He had watched as the new portable typewriter, the hi-fi record player, the portable sewing machine, and awkward tools were wrapped in our usable blankets and carefully placed into the steel drums we had purchased from bakeries after they were emptied of shortening.

“There will be plenty of bikes available in Africa,” said Dad as he clamped down the cover of a full barrel. He used a hammer to secure the steel rim.

“There more grownups ride bikes than kids.” Steve had seen lots of street pictures of African cities. “I want a bike, though.” He wanted, as much as we did, to cling to the familiar.

“Your favorite books . . . you've brought them all?” I reached for them. “We'll need all the books we can carry with us . . . no public libraries there . . . no bookstores close by." On top of the pile, I saw *The Little Engine That Could*, a book that would delight the little African boy, Joshua, and be left with him.

After the fourteenth barrel was filled and carried away as freight, which would be in port when we arrived in Africa, our apartment was bleak. The cupboards were empty except for necessities. We would be camping, so to speak, until the final day.

"The bike will just have to stick out of the trunk until we get home." My brother met Steve and me at the incoming train. Walt had stayed behind in Maywood to finish his summer school session while Steve and I went to spend a week in Minneapolis with Carl and Valborg. We had stayed with them before moving to the mission school.

"We haven't parted with it yet," I said apologetically. "Steve likes your neighborhood and wanted his bike."

The following week I attended a missionary conference at Luther Seminary in St. Paul. During those three days I visited with returned missionaries, gathering varied impressions. I was consciously being prepared for the worst regarding living conditions and inconveniences overseas, especially in Africa. "You'll have to boil all your drinking water," I was told, "and you'll be lucky if you have electricity for a few hours in the evenings when the generator works."

I realized that until now the thing that bothered me most was just the opposite: the deadening effect of too much prosperity, causing finer sensibilities to become numb or sluggish. If there is to be discomfort and inconvenience, or even hardship, it can be salutary.

Lately in the urban rush, I had a feeling Marangu on Mount Kilimanjaro would yield this kind of satisfaction. I sensed that what I valued most was still ahead, not left behind.

"The last of our luxuries. It's like parting with an old friend," I said as we watched the car salesman drive off in our red Oldsmobile. Walt had returned from Maywood driving our car, its last trip in our behalf.

"I still have my bike," said Steve as if to stave off nostalgia for the moment.

"Not for long. But I promised we would trade it in for a battery radio. How about that?" Dad put his hand on Steve's shoulder.

"Great," Steve replied without enthusiasm.

August 4, 1959, we were on our way, flying for the first time in our lives. We were flying on Northwest Airlines from Minneapolis to New York. With seatbelts fastened, we waited for liftoff. Would this aircraft with all its weight actually rest on the airwaves, no earth beneath? Indeed we did ascend . . . through the gray clouds, then through pure white clouds until we came into sunshine, radiant sunshine! How like the Ascension of Our Lord: up through the white clouds into brilliant light! I continued looking down into the abundance of clouds, seeing crevices and mountains, as it were, deep and high, but never hard, only as cotton batting is as one piece severs from another. How easily we had come through them! I knew now what was on the other side of thick clouds. I have always been inspired when flying.

6

August 1959, Tanganyika

Arriving in East Africa, I forgot all about cancer. It was as if I had never had such an experience. There was nothing here to remind me; this was a totally different world, Nairobi, Kenya. I was filled with wonder. My fellowmen were black; I had known they would be. Now I was among them. This new continent opened to us as we journeyed by car south into Tanganyika. We had our first glimpse of the wild savannah with its red soil, acacia trees, huge ant hills; a giraffe nibbling in the treetops. We came upon gazelle, wildebeest, and zebra grazing together in deep savannah grass, and we stopped to let a herd of thirty or more baboons cross the road in front of us.

At a rustic hotel in a place called Namanga, we stopped for a meal. We were served curry soup in which carrots, onions, and black, unappetizing flecks were floating. My bowl had an ugly brown crack from its center to the edge; our waiters were barefooted.

After eating, we took time to walk around the grounds. No bird we saw could we name. Insects and bright-colored lizards startled us. Trees, flowering vines, grass, and rock formations, all were as nothing we had ever known. A strange damp fragrance clung everywhere. Bird calls intermingled with the piercing hum of a million insects. Only the sky was familiar: clear blue with the white billowy clouds of a summer day.

We reached Marangu, our destination, after climbing five miles up the side of Mount Kilimanjaro. Surprisingly, the village was nowhere to be seen! All the homes were tucked out of sight on small plots under the broad leaves of banana trees.

We didn't see the campus either, as we drove along the narrow road lined with tall, vine-covered trees, until we turned up a steep driveway where we were confronted with a two-story stone building, Marangu Teacher Training College. Around the clearing were other stone buildings, evidently faculty houses and dormitories. Would we be settling here? There was something ancient about these buildings, built in the last century by German missionaries, since Tanganyika was originally a German colony. It seemed we were stepping back in history.

We first occupied a quaint stone cottage, nicknamed by past occupants as the "Three Bears' House," which was set aside for newcomers who would study Swahili and receive informal orientation around campus. We found ourselves among two Norwegian families, an American couple, and three single women, one a teacher and the other two nurses at the local hospital. We next moved into the "Big House," a vine-covered two-story, twelve-room mansion with four upstairs bedrooms opening onto a balcony where at night we could watch the brilliant moon and stars and at daybreak the sun rising far down on the savannah. The house was surrounded by exotic shrubs such as hibiscus, gardenia, poinsettia, and oleander. The yard was enclosed by an evergreen hedge ten feet high. Never had I dreamed of living in such a place! (It had its inconveniences, but I won't go into that.)

Walt and I began our teaching assignments at the beginning of the school year in January of 1960. Before that we came to appreciate the young male students by involving ourselves in chapel and Sunday services, special programs, and soccer games. So when classes began, we recognized individuals rather than simply a crowd of look-alike people as they had been at first. In my English classes, I found them eager and personable, a delightful discovery.

I had not shared my cancer experience with any of my new found friends in our campus community, congenial and caring though they were. There was no need; it was in the past until one day . . .

We had found a convenient swimming hole near us, at the foot of a waterfall, that was part of a stream that rushed down the mountain. The refreshing water from a melting glacier above brought us there on hot afternoons. One day Jan—her husband was the chaplain—Liz, one of the nurses, and I set out on the trail toward the falls. We wore our swimsuits under housecoats because females revealing legs in shorts, or even wearing pants, offended the populace. At the site was a convenient dressing room enclosed by two huge boulders with a tree branch for a roof, should there be onlookers from the trail above.

After our swim, we ate sandwiches and cookies Jan had made, then went to our shelter and housecoats.

"You've got a scar," whispered Jan.

"Mastectomy," I replied.

"No kidding!"

This exchange caught Liz's attention, and I hurried

to close my wrap. Sensing I didn't want to be a conversation piece, Liz continued drying her hair with a towel. Silently we wrapped our wet suits in towels and started back.

As we climbed the bank up to the path, I heard an echo; it was Gracie from months ago: "You keep an eye on it." I would waste no time.

"Liz, will you stop in a minute? I have something to show you," I announced as we reached the entrance through our hedge.

I led her into our bathroom and tossed off my housecoat. The mirror above the washbowl, the only one in the house, was too high for me to see more than my face.

"Take a look here," I said, tracing my way up the scar. "There is a stitch here I was told to watch." My finger landed on the spot and a wave of anxiety ran through me. It was certainly bigger—bean-size now!

Liz took her time. Since she was as competent as any general practitioner at her post here, we all trusted her with our health problems.

"You know what? I think you should have Dr. P. take a look at this. It is more than a stitch."

Dr. P. was a British doctor in Moshi, a city of several thousand inhabitants with a large population of Europeans, twenty-five miles down the mountain and to the east. I wasted no time getting to his office. In what was more like a cluttered kitchen than a medical center, I met a man, padding around in his bedroom slippers, who didn't look at all like a doctor. After a brief examination, Dr. P. recommended that I go to the hospital in Nairobi to have the nodule excised. "I will make an appointment for you with Dr. B.," he said. "You will also be given an x-ray, and their lab will report what they find."

This was no small matter, going the long distance to Nairobi for what seemed to me such a simple procedure. We arranged to be gone two days, or more if need be, causing quite a stir; trips to Nairobi didn't happen often.

The excision was simple; Dr. B. and his staff accomplished it without a hitch. Returning to his office, I was shown my x-ray and told it was free of any involvement.

"We will call Dr. P. in Moshi if your nodule turns out positive. He has connections with the Middlesex Hospital in London should you need radiation. That may not be the case, but his contacts there could prove valuable."

"Am I free to go?" I asked.

"Yes, indeed. Your prognosis is good, in my opinion. Whoever did your surgery did a wonderful job. In the States, I suppose?"

"Yes, State of Washington."

Dr. B. shook my hand. "Have a safe trip back to Tanganyika."

We started back about noon of the second day. Although we were in the midst of the rainy season, the main thoroughfare gave us no problems. The nodule was gone, and I was relieved. Even if it turned out to be positive, it was no longer a part of my body.

On our way through the savannah, we were suddenly slowed to a snail's pace by a lion walking in the middle of the road! No, she wasn't moving for us—she sensed that she had the right-of-way. Was she returning to her pride? Was she lost? Or, perhaps out for an additional meal. Who were we to understand the wild? We simply crawled along behind her and watched. She moved her head from side to side, peering as she went, her long tail curled enough to reveal its tufted end. I had seen tame cats moving like this. As quickly as she appeared, she was lost to us on the roadside.

"Look, she's following us!" Walt caught sight of her in the rearview mirror.

She was coming, all right, but soon she stopped and we lost sight of her standing in the road. Africa was expanding my concept of the unknown, the mysterious, the uncertain, and indeed of surprises. It wasn't frightening really; it called forth wonder and faith in God, the Eternal, the Creator of all, whose *thoughts are not our thoughts*, as the Psalmist says.

The assurance Dr. B. gave relieved my anxiety about cancer recurrence, and I devoted myself to teaching. English as a second language was a challenge for me. I marveled at my students, especially with regard to their self-esteem. No one put himself down, or anyone else for that matter. They were not competitors. They were open to what was to be mastered and never doubted their ability to do it. I found this refreshing, decent, and human, in contrast to attitudes prevailing at home.

One morning as I walked from our house to the chapel door, Johasi, our school secretary, rushed around the corner to meet me.

"Good morning," he said, coming to a sudden halt in front of me.

"Good morning, Johasi," I replied. No African

would begin a conversation without first a greeting, no matter how urgent the situation might be.

"I have a telephone message for you, Mrs. Gilseth," he said, handing me a written memo. "We received it about twenty minutes ago." He looked at his watch.

"Thank you." He felt himself dismissed and left. By most standards, telephone service to our school left something to be desired. There was only one telephone, and that was in the office. Messages were rare and difficult to negotiate, and we got along surprising well by using the mail. I had grown very content without the intruding phone.

Even before reading the note, I suspected it was something I didn't want to hear. Dr. P. was the caller. He had received the pathological report from Nairobi and wanted me to come to his office as soon as possible to discuss it. My heart sank. He wouldn't have bothered if the report had been negative.

The next day, Saturday, I went into Moshi with the school car and its driver, a routine weekly trip to bring back groceries and mail. I found Dr. P. at his home and sensed he was waiting for me. I would need radiation on my left chest wall, the sooner the better. No such service was available in East Africa. It would have to be Johannesburg, South Africa, or London. He could make arrangements for me with doctors he knew at the Middlesex Hospital in London. Time would not be wasted; he was sure they would take me right away. How long would I be gone? Five to six weeks at the most.

When I returned to campus, Walt said, "Perhaps this means we should go home to the States."

"Oh no," I objected, "not that. Why can't I just go to London and have done what needs to be done and then come back? Why should this be any different from a dental appointment—no fun but it has to be done? Besides, this can't wait. Who knows how long it would take to set up an appointment with doctors at home?"

"You mean you would go alone?"

"Why not? I'm a big girl."

"I could go with you. I'm sure arrangements could be made."

"It's bad enough to have one of us gone from the faculty without the both of us. And Steve comes home from school in another week. He'll need his dad."

The matter was settled between us. It wasn't, however, among our neighbors who, on hearing the news, had gathered in a small knot in our yard. "You can't go all alone! One of us could certainly accompany you," said one of the well-meaning Norwegian women.

"Wouldn't it be better to return to the States for such treatment?" was the concern of the Americans.

"London is not a frightening place." Liz stood up to the opposition. "I took my midwifery course at that very hospital. I'll be stopping off there on my furlough trip home in a couple of weeks." She nodded my way. "I'll look you up if you are still there." Not surprisingly, she had the last word.

"You're a brave woman," said our mission financial secretary as we stopped at his office in Moshi to relay our plans. "Your best bet is to have plenty of cash with you. You can always return to us what you don't spend. Those of us concerned about you can at least rest assured that you have ample means."

I smiled at him. "I am most grateful. I plan to stay at the YWCA, but if that doesn't work out, my lodging may cost me more." I watched him count denominations of British pound notes, becoming astonished at how much he intended to give me.

"There you are and may God go with you," he said, handing me a heavy brown envelope.

"Thank you so much." I shook his outstretched hand. "They do speak English there," I ventured, trying to keep matters lighthearted.

With my purse stuffed with British pounds and my referrals from Dr. P., we were again on our way north across the savannah to Nairobi. We were slowed to a halt again, not by a lion this time or a herd of baboons dashing across, but by a Maasai morani (youth—warrior class) and his herd of humpbacked cattle. He seemed to be the only herdsman, although the cattle were numerous. He stood in the middle of the road, directly in front of our windshield, and with his hand waved his animals across, although he was carrying a stick as well as a spear. A very handsome specimen he was, with his long braided strands of hair fluffed up with red ocher, the earth-colored makeup of the Maasai, together with the extravagant beaded earrings that hung from his slashed earlobes and the beaded flop that hung as a bang on his forehead. He wore a red rectangular cloth wrapped around his body, fastened with a tied knot on his left shoulder. His whole body was painted ocher, and his garment shared its grime. He escorted his cows; he didn't hurry them, therefore they were extremely docile. This crossing would take awhile.

Suddenly I felt a strong impulse to turn my head to the side. Two Maasai women were standing just outside our open window, staring in to satisfy their curiosity.

"Jambo," I said.

They responded simply with a laugh, showing beautiful white teeth. I decided they weren't laughing at me, this must be their way of greeting.

Both women had shaved heads, which, in their culture, designated them as married. Both wore cowhide skirts and drab brown shawls across their shoulders, covering their breasts. They wore beaded collars the size of dinner plates and earrings that dangled from pierced holes in the top of their ears. We continued smiling at each other. I wondered about their children. Where did they live—far from here? They had simply appeared from nowhere: a total surprise, another instance of my expanded unknown.

"They didn't reach out to beg," I told Walt as we finally got on our way. "They had dignity. Why should they envy me?"

"Not yet," was his reply and I knew he was right.

I waved once more at Walt high up on the observation deck at the Nairobi Airport, before climbing the steep metal ladder into my plane. Clinging desperately to my belongings, I groped my way along the aisle, searching for the number of my seat. Finally I settled in when suddenly I was seized with acute claustrophobia. I was flying out, leaving security behind! I broke out in a cold sweat. I groped for some rationale to quell the rush of dread. I sat in the very last seat in the section, and there was no window. The other seats had windows. Furthermore, a complete wall was at my back—I was indeed trapped. Soon a gentleman came and sat beside me. He was on his way home to London, after being away from his family for six months. Neither of us liked this seat, but I now had someone to share my misgivings. They soon faded.

I took out reading material carefully chosen for this long block of time. We had all been reading *Naught for Your Comfort,* by Trevor Huddleston—someone had given it up for me to carry along. South Africa and apartheid was a consuming concern of ours—continuity now with what I had left behind.

What lay ahead? I surprised myself at the courage I had—and it wasn't all pretense. I could only attribute it to that mysterious quality we call God's Grace . . . *I will fear no evil for Thou art with me.*

7
July 1960, London

London was a far different world from what I had left. Now at midmorning it was dark, the clouds hung low, and it was drizzling. The plane door swung out, and we climbed down and onto a shuttle bus that took us to the airport. Most of us stood huddled together, each of us hoping we were heading for the right building. We were lost in the mist.

The entry passport line was long, and I grew anxious. I looked for my seatmate, but he was gone; perhaps his family had met him. Finally at the window, I easily answered the routine questions, then took a taxi to the YWCA. We moved through the streets with me not used to seeing traffic moving forward on the left. I was confused and fascinated. I might try a double-decker bus sometime.

"We're all filled here," announced the woman at the YWCA desk as I set my suitcase down and approached her.

"I was counting on staying here," I replied. I was tired and tried not to sound helpless.

"You're an American. New to the city?"

"Yes. I am here from East Africa. I have a medical referral to Middlesex Hospital. Not far from here, is it? I hope to stay in the vicinity."

"Would you mind taking a room in a private flat?" She studied me for a moment. "I know of a place in Red Lion Square just a few blocks from here. You could leave your bags here and check it out."

Someone was caring; I was not out in the street. "Thank you," I said, coming closer.

She drew a map on a scratch pad as she explained where to go. This would be the private residence of an elderly woman named Mrs. King, who had one spare room and would let it out as bed and breakfast. "Be sure you tell her I sent you and give her this note. She takes only referrals from us." She came around, picked up my bags, and carried them into her office. "She will look you over before she decides to take you. Don't let that worry you. If she still wants to let the room, I think you're in."

Having found a plastic rain bonnet in my coat pocket, I set out into the London drizzle. This turn of events was baffling, but as I had discovered lately, the unknown could yield surprises. I reached an obscure entrance off the street and lifted the knocker.

After what seemed long enough to indicate there was no one at home, the door was opened by a bent little woman with a bed of hair piled loosely on top of her head. She had broad temples and a prominent, straight nose. With sharp eyes she engaged me.

"You have a room to let?" I dug for the referral in my purse and handed it over.

After she had studied the note, she lifted her head again and fixed her eyes on me. "You're an American. Umm. Come in, come in. What brings you to London?" She escorted me into a narrow, dark entry.

"I came from East Africa for medical treatment at Middlesex Hospital. I am a teacher in Tanganyika."

This sounded unreal to me, and I wondered what she would make of it. She led me to a door at the far end of the hallway and showed me into a small room. I saw, pushed against the wall, a single bed, which took up most of the room. It was covered with a snow-white spread, with a quaint Victorian doll propped against the pillow.

"Will this suit you?" she said, tossing out a hand as if to expand the area. "I will bring breakfast to your room each morning."

Then I noticed an overstuffed chair, a little table, and a chest of drawers. "Yes," I said, "this will be fine."

The sharp eyes brightened, she seemed pleased. "Let me show you the bath. It's just here on your right as we go into the hall." I followed through a door she opened for me. Most of the room was taken up with a hefty gray-white tub set upon a blue linoleum floor. Snow-white towels hung ready on the racks.

"Tell me an hour and a half ahead of time if you want a bath," she went on. "It takes that long to heat water."

"That's fine. I'll let you know." Coming directly from America, I might have resented this arrangement, but not now. In East Africa, we built a fire in a firebox under a cemented-in steel drum to heat our bath water.

"May I give you a cup of tea? You just arrived on a plane, you said?" asked Mrs. King.

"Yes, a cup of tea would be good," I replied without hesitation. "I was on the plane most of the night."

We walked past her small sitting room, where I noticed a parakeet in a cage, and into her tiny kitchen. She sat me at a small table covered with a linen lunch cloth. She brought two cups, a teapot, and a plate of shortbread cookies, which the British refer to as biscuits, to the table and seated herself opposite me.

"What's going to happen at Middlesex Hospital, if you don't mind my asking?" She reached for the teapot and filled our cups.

"I'm about to have cobalt radiation. A malignant lump has been removed from a scar in my chest wall. The doctors have decided I should have radiation." I took a sip of tea.

"Cancer?" She put down her cup and looked at me a long moment. "And you're here all by yourself—you poor dear!"

No, I decided, she wasn't just a busybody; I chose to accept her interest and concern. I wasn't excused until she heard all the details. She wanted to know about my prognosis, my teaching job in Tanganyika, my family, and why we were so far from home. Before I left she assured me that if there was anything she could do for me, just let her know. Did I like milk at bedtime—a hot-water bottle?

I returned to the YWCA feeling the warmth of this newly-made friend. Before picking up my bags, I tried to call the hospital on a pay phone, but found it very confusing. The coins I had didn't seem to fit, and I couldn't interpret the buzzing signals. Finally I decided to go to the hospital in person the first thing Monday morning, this being Friday afternoon with nothing open on weekends.

"Good morning," said Mrs. King, entering with a tray. "Sunday morning we serve kippers for breakfast together with our eggs, and today, marmalade and muffins."

"Thank you," I responded feebly. I scarcely grasped

what her knock on the door was all about, to say nothing of having breakfast in bed.

"Perhaps you would prefer coffee to tea in the mornings?" She set the tray down on the bedside table. "What I will do is get a jar of instant coffee and bring you hot water. This morning I can only offer you tea."

"Tea is fine, though, as you said, I do prefer coffee," I replied as I raised myself on my elbows. "Thanks so much. I'm sure I will enjoy my breakfast."

She turned abruptly and left. She was a businesswoman who maintained a bed and breakfast. By no means would I be neglected. I should have responded to the idea of kippers but was too slow coming forth with anything. Fish for breakfast?

I had two days to spend before Monday. I hung my clothes in a large wardrobe that I had mistaken for one of the four walls. I placed my books on top of the chest of drawers and used the drawer space for my meager belongings. After settling in, I went for a walk around the neighborhood, getting acquainted with my surroundings. I stopped at a telephone booth. With Sunday coming up, I had in mind to contact what was described to me, by friends before I left, as the only Lutheran church in London. I got out my coins to experiment with the telephone as I had done the day before. After struggling with a disconnected number, I finally got the church office and reached an American voice happy to tell me what worship services and activities they had to offer.

Venturing beyond Red Lion Square, I found a street with several shops. Why not splurge and buy a new dress? New shoes? Now that I was in London, my East Africa clothes had begun to feel tacky; I pictured myself going to church in the morning in new clothes. Why not?

"Yes, I am American." I acknowledged that fact every place I went, if not verbally, at least with a smile to break the ice as clerks looked at one another. Perhaps I was too self-conscious. Having bought a light dress and a pair of high-heeled shoes, I finished my shopping at a pharmacy where a very accommodating clerk wanted to talk.

"Don't be afraid to take the subway here in London. It's the best way to get around. That vast underground network was our air-raid shelter during the war." With his help I learned the subway linked me to famous sites that I must not fail to see. I listened intently. Tomorrow I would commute by subway to church.

The sun was shining and pigeons awaited hand-outs in Red Lion Square. After depositing my parcels and telling Mrs. King I wanted a bath, I returned to the Square with my letter-folio. I would write to Steve and compose silly limericks about pigeons and street scenes. I wasn't letting myself get lonesome, not yet. In my mind's eye, I saw my son's smile, and even heard a giggle at what his mother put into rhyme.

I saw a comic artist
With a piece of colored chalk
He was drawing on the street
Right where people walk.

His cap he put beside him
Hoping any minute
A passer-by would smile and nod
And put a penny in it

I found a small Italian restaurant in the vicinity and ordered dinner. I hoped it would suit me, since I needed a place for meals during my stay.

"I hear you are American." A hearty voice spoke my dialect, and a large woman arrived at my table, smiling broadly and ready to make my acquaintance.

"How could you guess?" I asked.

"I heard you order your meal. Mind my intruding?" She had a bright round face, gray eyes and red perm'd hair, not carefully groomed.

"Not in the least. Join me." She went back for her coffee cup and slid in opposite me. She was wearing a tan all-weather coat over a flowery dress. She reminded me of someone I knew, with whom I felt very comfortable, but I couldn't think of whom.

"Where in the States are you from?" she began the conversation as she settled in front of me.

"From Minnesota. I have just now come from Tanganyika, East Africa, where I am a teacher.

"What brings you to London?"

To this question I went into further detail than I had intended since, she, like Mrs. King, continued to probe me. "Here all alone—you're a brave woman!" she said, just like the rest had done, but with a difference—she seemed intent on doing something about it. She told me that she was from Pennsylvania and an ordained clergy person in the Congregational church. She was in London with a group of American students touring sites and doing study projects. "You say you hope to see your appointed doctor on Monday morning? I'll tell you what. Why don't we meet afterwards? I'll be anxious to hear what is about to happen. My students and I often eat at a little restaurant near that hospital—there is a small cove where we meet just to talk and compare notes. You could meet us there—pretend we are family. What do you say?"

"I say yes. How very thoughtful of you!" I could hardly believe what I was hearing. "But I might be delayed—I have no idea when I will be finished."

"We have much to discuss among ourselves. We'll be there."

After she jotted down the name of the restaurant for me, we parted and I carried her warmth with me. I wasn't necessarily brave; God must have sent her to me. I tried to remember whom she reminded me of—it was surely someone I dearly loved from home.

I assumed the water was warm when I entered the flat. As I prepared to bathe, I shook the wrinkles out of my new dress and hung it in the wardrobe. I looked at the shoes and saw how ridiculous they were; I would never walk around in these in East Africa. Closing my bathrobe, I stole into the bathroom and closed the door. I turned on the faucets—nice warm water. I hunched my right foot over the edge of the huge tub and slowly sank down in comfort, ready to sit a long time. This was nice. Wool-gathering, I focused on Steve's reading the limericks I had sent him. I smiled again as I had sitting on the park bench. I was working at protecting him from anxiety over his mother who had left for London to go to the Middlesex Hospital because of cancer. Sending letters with little caricatures might be another thing I could do.

But how could I protect him from my death—losing his mother! Hadn't I had a recurrence? Didn't that always mean imminent death? A wave of panic ran through me! Fiercely I rubbed soap into the washcloth to abate the emotional impact. *Wait! This minute everything is okay.* I told myself, *Panic is never legitimate—*

calm down! Use your God-given good sense; that's what Kierkegaard did when terror struck him. Slowly I covered myself with fragrant suds. I drew more warm water from the faucet and slid deeper into the tub. Once again I was calm, at least for now.

Jacob wrestled. Job cried out. I was headed for a night like theirs as I crawled into Mrs. King's bed, in a city far from home. *Oh, God are you going to let me die? You must know that my husband and son need me—they cannot do without me—it is irresponsible for me to leave them—you must be on our side—I've just begun to live, as we say, at the age of forty—it's illogical—it's—it's—don't you understand, God?*

He was hiding His face; it was no use. The bed bounced as I made a swift swing around.

Who did Charlotte remind me of? She said her name was Charlotte, didn't she? I would see her again after my trip to the doctor. The thought was like a hand on my shoulder; it felt good. I continued to picture her face until I fell asleep.

I woke Sunday to fish for breakfast, smoked kippers with my eggs. Plenty of coffee, Nescafé instant, to be made with the hot water brought in a teapot. I had planned my day, no time for idle worry. I put on my new dress, the high-heeled pumps and a tiny straw hat with a wisp of veil. I was going to church, and I would take the tube.

The vast subway station described to me the day before was nearly deserted at this hour on Sunday morning. I was glad when the rushing subway train came to a halt and the automatic doors swung wide open to accept me. Only two other passengers occupied this car. Not seeing the elevator (or lift, as the British call it) as I got off the train, I climbed a circular steel stairway for what seemed an incredibly long time until I reached the street. I breathed a sigh of relief after imagining what I might have encountered there.

I found the church easily and joined an adult class for visitors to the city. Here I met Margorie, a sprightly young woman with whom I would enjoy the museums and concert halls of London. She was an organist from Wisconsin, studying for a degree in church music. We became friends for the duration of my stay, beginning this first Sunday after church when we had lunch together and visited Hyde Park.

As I received the Eucharist during the communion service, I again searched for my lost God. I had a step to take—that one step more that Kierkegaard wrote about in his *Purity of Heart.* " . . . go with God to God, continually take that one step more."

Sobering thoughts returned as I boarded a bus from Hyde Park back to Red Lion Square after an entertaining afternoon with my vivacious new friend, Margorie. The crucial hour of Monday morning was drawing closer. There was something about my venture now that was as unreal as Narnia in the book Steve and I read together: *The Lion, the Witch and the Wardrobe,* by C. S. Lewis. "Was the lion Aslan safe?" the children had asked. "No, of course he is not safe, but he is good. Trust him! Trust him!"

All was quiet and dark as I used my key to let myself into Mrs. King's flat. I remembered my recent panic as I made my way past the bathroom door. As I entered my room, however, I found a bowl of fruit and two Cadbury bars on top of the chest of drawers, another of Mrs. King's kind gestures. I ate a banana. Although it was not quite bedtime, I changed into my robe and sat in the overstuffed chair.

Yes, I had that step to take. *Trust Him! He is wiser than you are—infinite wisdom. Yes, I trust Your goodness. I consent to die if You will promise to be with me. I guess, mostly, I feel unsafe, frightened. I want to will what You will. Let me leap into Your arms!*

The next moment was ecstatic: *Peace that passeth all understanding!* Could this last? Could it?

"Good luck to you, my dear," called Mrs. King from her kitchen, sensing I was on my way to the hospital.

"Thank you. I'll be back before long, I hope." I shut the door behind me. I walked the four blocks and climbed the long wide steps into what indeed looked like the prestigious place I had heard so much about. I received immediate attention, as a result of my references, and sat only a short while in a little waiting room.

"Your doctor, my old friend, thrives in East Africa. I don't think he will ever return," began this doctor who, I was to learn later, was the most prestigious of British cancer specialists. "I suppose that country can grow on you."

"I have lived there for less than a year and am quite taken with it," I replied. My mind focused on what his diagnosis would be.

"The surgeon who did your mastectomy did a beautiful job," he said upon concluding his examination.

That again—I guess I should be grateful. He seated himself on a stool with casters and rolled himself to the desk. He shuffled through my papers and jotted further notes.

"We will give you a course of cobalt," he said, now quite prepared to explain what I had come all the way to London to know. "I wouldn't prescribe deep x-ray over the whole area, just around the fresh scar. You will come every day, five days a week, omitting Saturday and Sunday, for twenty-four doses. Each treatment takes seven minutes. We will give you plenty of notice when the time comes to leave for Nairobi since plane reservations are sometimes difficult to get. You may have some soreness, depending on the condition of your skin. We will start you off today. It seems I can get you in right away."

I left the hospital in a hurry, Charlotte's scribbled note, naming the restaurant where we had agreed to meet, in hand. She was there, all right. I barely entered when she rushed to meet me. We embraced.

"Things are working out," I hastened to say. "I got to see my doctor right away."

"Well, good for you. I'm so glad to hear it. Come and meet my friends."

I was drawn to a table strewn with notebooks and empty coffee cups around which sat three youths, unmistakably American. I was delighted to join them as another chair was brought for me.

"Pastor Charlotte has told us all about you. Now tell us what happened this morning," said one young man as I settled in with them.

"Yes, do." Charlotte looked at me as if to say, *That's why you're here.*

"The doctor doesn't think I need deep x-ray over my whole chest wall, just over the new scar." I was feeling comfortable enough to continue. "I had my first treatment today. A circle was drawn around my scar as I lay under a machine in the radiation room. A curious little box, about two cubic inches in size and attached to a vacuum hose, was placed over the circle.

When the machine was turned on, pebbles rattled into the box and remained there for the seven-minute duration until the vacuum drew them back through the hose. This is going to happen to me daily until I have completed twenty-four doses. Not bad, huh?"

"Only seven minutes a day in the hospital?" My listeners were attentive.

"Right, lots of time to enjoy London." I wasn't sure whether it was the audience or the news I brought that gave me the most joy, but I certainly was on Cloud Nine.

"Museums, concerts, plays—you'll have a ball." More than one were speaking now.

"I might even make it to Stratford on Avon!" I exclaimed.

Before leaving, Charlotte and I made a date to meet again after she returned from a trip out of town.

Four days later, after hearing my footsteps in the hall, Mrs. King followed me to my room.

"See what came in the post. Nine blue airforms from Africa. Your friends certainly remember you." She handed me my prize.

"Thank you. I must say I am rewarded for waiting." As I spoke, she nodded and smiled. She left me alone to read them.

There were letters from everyone, including six students. One wrote, "Don't worry about your son Steven; we are his companions."

8

April 1966, Resolving Culture Shock

The sickeningly-sweet odor was still in my nostrils and crystallized in the back of my head. It lingered on my tongue like stale wine.

"Feeling bad? You received ether as your anesthetic. It's not used much anymore, but that's all our anesthetist had to offer." A nurse with a broad smiling face was looking down at me. "We put some medicine for nausea in your IV. It should help some."

I could only respond with a feeble smile. Yes, Dr. T. told me last evening it would be ether. Had this been Africa, I wouldn't have been at all surprised, but here in Marshall, Minnesota? My surgery was urgent, he said. It might take a week to get another anesthetist. He planned to remove my remaining ovary (one had been removed years ago because of a cyst) to rid my body of estrogen, which causes tumors. A week ago he removed a tumor from my chest wall, which proved to be malignant. Now he was taking prompt action. He had been treating me with estrogen for menopause and with chagrin quickly took me off that medication.

I continued to look into the kind face of the nurse. *Where had I been? So far away and so helpless! Now I was safe.* I wanted to embrace her as if she were my mother. I smiled again and said, "Thank you."

"You've been thanking me ever since you returned from surgery. I feel very much appreciated." She laughed, wanting me to laugh with her.

How could I begin to tell her how it was? I had inhaled an icy fragrance that caused a huge kaleidoscope of many bright moving bits of color to appear. I felt myself in the center of it. I was startled as it moved swiftly to a great distance, becoming pointed as a needle, growing smaller as it went. Finally like a door slamming shut, it was no more—gone! Long gone! Until now as wave after wave of nausea swept over me. The crystal hold that the sweet odor held on my head was loosening. The stale wine was escaping my tongue.

The nurse was standing by, holding the sputum dish. "Here, lie back again." She put the dish aside, fluffed my pillow, and wound down the bed.

"I'm very tired."

"That's the way—just sleep it off."

I trust Dr. T.—the thought brushed again through my consciousness. It brought me back to last evening when he restitched the incision that had gaped open because I carelessly reached for a book on the top shelf of my classroom cupboard. For the past two years, we have lived in the town of Cottonwood, twenty-three miles from Marshall. I teach English, and Walt is the elementary principal.

"You're a very active woman," he said, having taken care to deaden the flesh where the needle would penetrate. I relaxed somewhat, but not enough to handle conversation, let alone to acknowledge compliments. "Do you know the story of Elijah—from the Old Testament Book of Kings?" He stopped and looked at me for a moment.

"I believe I do. Why?"

"The music society I belong to is working on Mendelssohn's oratorio, *Elijah.* Do you know it?"

"I've heard of it, that's all."

While he stitched, he related with reverence the oratorio's content, the dramatic story told in aria and chorus. I listened like a child, forgetting the in and out of the needle and thread. I wanted him to stay when it was over. "See you in the morning," he said with an assuring smile. Tomorrow came and he did the surgery.

Back in my room, I was safe. Since my nurse had encouraged me to sleep, I stretched my legs and took a deep, clean breath. I enjoyed being awake a while.

In the semidarkness, I let my mind wander and thought again about Elijah, for I was like Elijah, I didn't want the image of him to leave. Elijah was sad and alone, staying in a cave. The voice of the Lord spoke to him, saying, "What are you doing here, Elijah?" Elijah replied, "It is enough now, Lord, take away my life . . . . " The Lord said, "Go, return on your way, and when you arrive there will be work for you to do." An angel fed him, giving him strength for the journey. Like Elijah, I needed strength for the challenge. As I let him go, a cloud took him, or was it a chariot?

I was suddenly in my American literature classroom. I recognized Robert Frost:

> The woods are lovely dark and deep,
> But I have promises to keep,
> And miles to go before I sleep,
> And miles to go before I sleep.

"Do you want a bit to eat? Supper trays are coming up."

"I'll try," I said, and heard Walt's firm footsteps in the hall. He came in wearing the bright-colored shirt I had made for him while still in Africa. He must like that shirt.

"Well, here you are awake and ready to eat! You were out a long time." He took my hand and smiled at me. Had I realized before what a wonderful smile he has?

"I have been far away. I finally came back—and now you have come." I felt as though I babbled. The tray came and my bed was raised to meet the table rolled in front of me.

"It's chicken soup, I believe," said Walt as he lifted the lid from a serving dish. "Crackers, buttered bread—and what do you know, Jell-O—red Jell-O!"

The smell of chicken soup struck a raw nerve. "I'll eat the Jell-O."

He quickly covered the soup. "Is that all?"

"All I need right now." I began to melt tiny bites of Jell-O in my mouth.

"Everything is fine at home. Our elkhound has taken to wandering again, but the whole town knows that Loki is not dangerous and rather welcomes the sight of him. Not bad to live in a small town."

Returning from distance space, I slowly began to focus on what Walt was telling me.

"Mrs. C. is holding forth in your classes. I think she likes substituting for you. She asked me how long you would be gone. She wants to send written greetings from your students one of these days."

"How is Steve?" I asked.

"He and Bud are out on their bikes every spare moment now that the ice and snow have disappeared."

I spooned the slippery Jell-O into my mouth until at last I had enough.

"Want to lie back down again?" Walt rolled the table away. "I'll content myself with today's paper while you snooze again."

I watched him get comfortable in the armchair by the window. Did he wear that wild-colored shirt to please me? He knew how hard it was for me to accept the idea of not returning to Tanzania. We could have gone back and continued work on the religion curriculum for middle schools, which had been my primary task in our third and fourth years there. However, as far as teaching was concerned, we had pretty well worked ourselves out of the job as many African students were returning from education abroad to step into teaching positions. And that was as it should be. How would we break into the school system here at home if we had been out of the country for many years and become that much older? It was the right decision, there was no question about that.

Walt and I always work things out together. It was good to have him sitting there by the window. And he bothered to tell me that Loki had taken to wandering, and people accepted him wherever he went. Now in my mind's eye, I saw Roger, our African Ridgeback, standing in the driveway the morning we left, wondering how long we would be gone. He knew we always returned. But not this time. The decision not to return was soul-wrenching. We had made it together, Walt and I. But even today, although I know in my head it was right, I still feel pain. Like Roger, I am still standing in the driveway.

I heard the rustling of newsprint and hoped he wouldn't get up and leave. We are carried by a restless tide, these days, fast pace, always on the move. He settled again. We returned in August of 1963 to Lynden, Washington, and at the request of our mission board, we accepted invitations to speak and show slides at various churches in the area. I remember the agony of dressing up in the new styles: short tight miniskirts with tiny spike-heeled dress shoes—no more a simple blouse and dirndl skirt with wide flat shoes and ankle socks. Our audiences didn't take us seriously, they preferred our animal slides and exotic shots of the Maasai. Steve and I would wait for Walt's comments on the ostrich, "big drumsticks," then look at each other with a concealed giggle—he said it every time.

We left Washington State in early December, crossing the Rockies in a Volkswagen Bug, the same kind of car we drove in Africa. After spending Christmas with our folks in Minneapolis, we proceeded to Maywood, Illinois in time for second semester where we were to complete the master's programs we each had begun four years earlier. We stayed in the same apartment house on the seminary campus, Walt commuting to Concordia University, River Forest, where he eventually earned his degree, while I studied on the Maywood campus.

When school was out, Steve and I left for a Lutheran Bible Camp on Lake Okoboji in northwest Iowa, leaving Walt at Maywood to finish his courses. We were assigned to the camp by our mission board as "Missionaries in Residence" for the summer, with a new group of campers due each week. We decked a table in our assigned barracks with our ebony carvings brought back from Africa and hung colorful *kanga*, the colorful rectangular cloths African women wrapped around themselves as a garment, around the walls. We worked our slide showings for three different age groups. We swam every afternoon, as it turned out to be a hot summer, and Walt, when he wasn't on the road applying for a job for the coming school year, visited on weekends.

"You look sad," said a woman next to me at an evening bonfire. "I will pray for you."

I was not aware that my anxiety about getting settled for the coming school year was showing. However, I was grateful for her show of love.

The next day Walt arrived. "I have an interview for us at Cottonwood, Minnesota, just north of here. You must come with me tomorrow.

"For us?" I asked.

"There are two vacancies, one English, the other social studies. It's the best prospect I've seen yet."

So I left my little choir with Steve as they beat the African drum and sang Swahili songs, and we found our way into western Minnesota. Cottonwood was a clean little town. It could be home, we thought, as we drove around, seeking the school building.

"You have credentials for being an elementary principal, and I need one badly!" the superintendent began speaking before we were seated. "Social studies teachers are easy to come by, but not the elementary principal I need—doubtful I could find one before September." He motioned to us to sit and dropped into the chair behind his desk. "What's more, I need an English teacher, also not too easily found. I have looked over your papers and am ready to offer you the positions."

We looked at each other. Elementary principal, had it ever entered the picture? We left Cottonwood that day with signed contracts. As we drove through the camp entrance and passed the site of evening bonfires, I remembered my friend whom I had known so briefly. Her prayer had been answered.

The paper rustled again, being folded and tossed aside. "Been sleeping? You have more color in your face," Walt said as he drew close to the bed.

"Not much, I guess. Consciousness brings with it a string of things. I simply let it all come."

"Visiting hours are over. I'd better go," he said looking at his watch. "Rev. S. said he would drop in to see you tomorrow. He visits here Wednesday mornings, he told me. He will bring the Eucharist should you want it now during Holy Week."

"That's thoughtful of him," I replied, but without feeling. He could come if he wanted. "I hate to see you leave. I'll wait patiently until you get back. You have school tomorrow, I realize, but not on Friday. I'll see more of you then. Evenings? You'll be here?"

"I certainly will. And now get well. We need you." He bent over to kiss me. "Say your prayers and so will we." He disappeared as suddenly as he had come.

Left alone, I felt one of my frequent waves of depression returning. Pastor S. would be here in the morning. Why didn't I look forward to seeing him? He seemed absent in my presence. Indeed, he had a pastor's demeanor, dispensing caring in so many kind words that I failed to take him to heart. He wasn't too different from the rest of the congregation, or indeed from any of my own people since I returned from Tanzania. How could I make them understand that I had met people in Africa who were totally present with me, a stream of recognition flowing back and forth in every encounter—acceptance, trust. Oh, how I miss them! I hadn't resolved my loneliness, although two years had passed since I last saw any of them. Would time and its inevitable forgetfulness fade this wonderful taste of community and belonging from my consciousness? I hoped not!

Then Emily came to mind. We had just finished doing *Our Town*, by Thornton Wilder, in American literature class. I suddenly identified with that young woman who came back from the dead to relive her twelfth birthday.

"Oh, Mama, just look at me one minute as though you really saw me!" then finally exclaiming, "Oh, oh, it goes so fast we don't have time to look at one another . . . take me back up the hill!"

Heaven would be a place of total presence, everyone totally present for one another. I had caught a glimpse of a transcendent quality of life; I could count on it, it wouldn't be lost.

"I'm bringing you something for pain and to help you sleep." A new nurse was on duty. "But first a back-rub." She had me sit up while I soaked up the comfort of the rub, and she stayed long enough to fluff my pillow. After a shot was administered in my hip, she lowered the lights. "Sleep well and call us if you need us." She walked out, leaving the door slightly ajar.

I entered Christ Lutheran Church in Cottonwood, my home church now, thinking I was early as I looked around at the worshipers who had gathered this Sunday morning. They were all appropriately dressed for church attendance, and spread apart in the pews as if space were needed between people. I was getting used to this now, but found it so different from Nguruma, our congregation in Tanzania, where people always managed to slide in one more person. A bench for six would do for ten, no space between. Despite this there was always an overflow crowd along the walls or even outside by the open windows. I missed those who came in their rags, so to speak, and barefooted if need be, to be among the worshipers. I never saw the poor at Christ Lutheran, and I missed them. I chose a pew two-thirds of the way down, occupied by three other persons. From habit I was prepared to slide in farther should the need arise.

The organist in her white gown at the console of the recently installed pipe organ began her flawless prelude. I sensed the sanctuary filling up but was very surprised when an African woman with a plump infant moved into my pew. "Salaam," she whispered with a smile, expecting me to move even farther, causing the other three persons to move to the far end. Other women and girls in colorful *kanga* and *kitamba* (clothing) followed her until the pew was tightly occupied. Now I saw that the whole sanctuary was filling up with Africans, nodding and smiling, men on the left, women on the right. The choir members were sliding close together in their pews also as Africans joined them. Africans began finding room at the front when all the pews were full, sitting on the floor in a row in front of the first pews, then on the chancel steps and even on the steps mounting the pulpit. As I turned my head, I saw more comers along the outer aisle along the windows. They brought the odor of their cooking fires with them.

I grew uneasy. Would this be taken as an intrusion by the members of my church? I looked about for an answer. I saw signs of annoyance, shifting shoulders, at being expected to make room for the comers. Most refused eye-contact to accept a smile, a few responded through tight lips. I only had to wait until we began to sing! No need to share hymn books, the songs were fully known, except, of course, in another language. The men undergirded the melody by singing bass with firm voices while the women broke into alto and soprano. The harmony raised the hymn beyond amazement. Who was listening to the organ, as if it were required to furnish the total musical setting?

Would the service go on and on even as in Tanzania? I became aware that the choir had acquired new life. With wonder I heard an anthem I had taught the Marangu College Choir: "Light of Light Enlighten Me," by Bach. I vowed I'd never direct a choir after Marangu. None that I had ever directed before could reach their heights; Africans sang as easily as they breathed, and if there was no reason to sing, they would make one, at work camps, at athletic events, in their dorm rooms.

We marched to the chancel with our offering this morning, something we seldom did here, but always there. As I reached the end of my pew, moving to the front, I saw a familiar face—it was Immanueli, one of our students and my best tenor! "*Kwa Heri,* [good-bye] Mama Gilseth, even as you leave our country we shall meet again!"

"*Asanti sana* [thank you]," I replied feeling his glow, "*na Kwa Heri.*" I clung to his hand as long as I could, but we were holding up the crowd. These words were an echo of our farewells two years ago. Strange how they had come into the present.

"*Mwokozi Yetu* [Beautiful Savior]" was what I heard as a strange, familiar peace began to settle for me, here it was! Suddenly without warning the whole sanctuary spun like a kaleidoscope of many colors and we were lifted away; as to the point of a needle we made distance, great distance—

I awoke. The glow of my dream hung around a long time. Was this to be the resolution to my loneliness? These wonderful people had not gone away; I had just seen them. Whenever I worship they will be there.

It must soon be sunrise. I saw a touch of daylight at the window. I had slept through the whole night.

"We eat breakfast early around here," said a rise-and-shine voice. Another nurse was on duty ready to wake me. She set a wash basin before me and held a towel ready.

"Good morning," I said, surprised that my voice was actually cheery.

After the morning routine, I was robed and seated in a chair. "If it feels good being up, you may stay there as long as you like," my attending nurse said as she went out the door.

"Hello, there." Pastor S. had slipped through the open door. There he stood, wearing his clerical collar, waiting for recognition.

"Good morning, Pastor. Please come in and pull up a chair if you can find one."

"It's good to see you sitting up." He took my hand. "You're looking bright and perky this morning."

"I'm not complaining, but I'll be glad to be home."

"Here's our Sunday bulletin so you can keep up with us. We'll all be happy to have you back." He found himself a chair.

"Thank you." I watched him place his little black communion kit on the bed table before sitting down.

"You know, I dreamt about you last night, Pastor."

"Not too terrifying, I hope."

"You were conducting service from the altar in the chancel of our church in your robe, but you were not alone. Pastor Gabrieli of Nguruma Congregation, Tanzania, Africa, was beside you dressed in his white surplice and red stole. You two looked alike, except you were white and he was black. I do believe you read the Scripture lessons, but he conducted the liturgy. The musical setting throughout was in the Swahili language. It was exquisite! The church was full of worshipers, our own people, but also a host of African Christians who had come to worship with us. It was a wonderful experience for you; your face was radiant."

"That's very touching," said Pastor S.

"I only wish this might have been your dream as well as mine, so you could describe what this experience was like—hundreds of voices singing." I looked at him, wanting a reply.

"I'm glad you found me receptive. I guess that is all I can say to that."

I understood this was all he could say. "I'm ready to receive communion now," I said. "It is thoughtful of you to bring it, particularly now that it is Holy Week."

I felt better about him now. He had admitted his lack of my experience, it was not to be expected. I watched him open the mysterious little box. He found a tiny glass for the wine and filled it. He drew forth a wafer. *Take and eat, this is My Body . . .*

Elijah's angel was coaxing me, *Rise and eat; the journey is too much for you.* I wouldn't try to explain this allusion to Pastor S. That didn't matter now; I simply let him be God's messenger. He left after he had reverently closed the black kit; he had others to visit before the morning was over.

The journey: that must be reckoned with. I was preoccupied with what possibly lay before me even as I was coaxed to eat and sleep. I would have radiation at Northwestern Hospital in Minneapolis as soon as this was over. Would the absence of estrogen help keep tumors from showing up? Mrs. C. would take care of my classes until I returned. My English students were important to me. So were the eighth-graders who needed extra help in reading. The SRA boxes (Science Research Associates) of progressive lessons and programmed reading workbooks were beginning to pay off, and Steve was one of several who benefited. Time must be found for this enrichment to continue.

In late afternoon I heard Walt's footsteps in the hall. He was still wearing the wild-colored shirt—good for him!

"I have good news," he exclaimed.

"You do? I can't imagine."

"We received the federal Title One grant for your summer school project. Remember the effort you put into applying for that? Well, it's here! President Johnson's Great Society hits Cottonwood!"

"Return and I will show you what to do," the Lord said to Elijah.

9

November 1976, Learning from Another

"We're moving you to a room on the fifth floor this morning." A pleasant nurse had just recorded my vital signs. "It's time for you to leave intensive care. You're lucky. You'll like it much better there."

My last major surgery had occurred during Holy Week, ten years before in Marshall, Minnesota, when an ovary was removed. Now, as tumors continued to spread in my left chest wall requiring excision, a portion of my second rib had also been removed. I had been closely monitored for the last three days and the ever-gurgling drainage pump had been at my side.

In the fall of 1966, we had moved from Cottonwood to St. Charles, Minnesota, where Walt became principal of a large elementary school and I taught English in the local high school. Living close to Rochester's Mayo Clinic, I found dependable medical attention for my problem of recurring nodules. I've lost track of how many times one, two, or three grains have been excised, some at the clinic, but more often as an outpatient at Methodist Hospital. A couple of times tumors were so deeply embedded that I was put to sleep and kept overnight.

"I understand you're leaving intensive care this

morning," said the house chaplain, who seemed to appear out of nowhere. "I thought I might stop in to wish you well."

"Thank you." I was pleased to see him. "I have something to tell you. Usually recovery-room experiences are nothing to brag about, but not this time. At the moment I awoke, I saw myself at Palm Sunday worship in my church. The Sunday school children and I were doing choral reading with gusto. It was the Twenty-fourth Psalm, great for choral reading since it is question and answer.

> "Who is the King of Glory?
> The Lord, Strong and mighty,
> The Lord, mighty in battle.
> He is the King of Glory!

"As I became aware of where I was, I thought doctors and nurses would come running from all directions; but no one even noticed me."

"So you woke to the sound of children. That's remarkable!" He reached in his vest pocket for his copy of the New Testament with Psalms.

"Extraordinary to say the least! You'll read Psalm Twenty-four now?" What could be more appropriate to hear upon leaving the uncertainty of this room? While he read, the wheelchair escort entered and paused respectfully.

"May God go with you," he said. At the door he turned and faced me with a departing nod.

"Thank you," I said. Now the nurse stood beside me as the wheelchair was brought to the edge of my bed. "You'll have a roommate in room 506." She raised me to a sitting position on the side of the bed.

"I don't think I'll mind," I said, wondering why she needed to prepare me in advance. Having a hospital roommate would be a new experience for me. I guessed this woman had also had surgery, possibly for cancer. Patients with similar care needs would no doubt be on the same floor.

While I was helped into the wheelchair, someone gathered my belongings, books, four floral bouquets friends had sent, Kleenex and back-rub lotion along with my little suitcase. As we moved through the hall to the elevator, I felt like part of a parade—well-wishers waving at me. Coming out of the elevator, we passed a sunroom, bright as all outdoors. I hadn't seen daylight for days and wanted to linger, but there was no time for that.

When the wheelchair and cart stopped at room 506, I caught a glimpse of my roommate propped in an armchair by the window, asleep. She woke as the blinds were opened and smiled like a child at the bright sunshine, and then at me. It was a generous welcome. Then I realized my roommate had a visitor.

"Bessie, here's your new roommate." The voice was sugary. "This is Elizabeth Bailey," she told me, "and I am Agnes, her sister-in-law. I closed the drapes earlier because the sun was directly on her." The voice was apologetic.

This woman's broad face and muscular arms recalled the farm folk where I'd grown up. She gave the impression that she would do anything for her kin—even put out the sun itself, if necessary. But the light warmed Bessie; she had dozed off again.

Agnes then turned to me. Where was I from? Had I also had surgery? Bessie's former roommate had gone home that morning; she had had a hysterectomy and gotten along just fine. She hoped Bessie could go home for Thanksgiving. She'd had surgery for colon cancer, and her cancer had spread. Bessie was her husband's sister, and she would come to live with them now since she wouldn't be able to care for herself until she got stronger. Running up to the hospital was becoming a chore and some days she couldn't come until after six, since she worked in a laundry. And it was certainly getting cold. It was no fun getting around on those icy streets.

"Time to get you up on your feet." Two healthy, young women in white had suddenly entered, and their beaming presence was not to be ignored. Bessie opened her eyes as though she had already come to terms with what she must do. "Put your hands on the arms of your chair and raise yourself. That's right."

The blanket comforting the tired knees was pulled away and tossed on the bed. She was on her feet now, supported on both sides. They walked past the foot of my bed. I was proud of her. Swaggering in the arms of those who held her, she marched along, holding her head erect and her chin firm. I watched them go through the door. How far would they take her? I shuddered.

"Her strength doesn't seem to be returning; the cancer must be spreading." Agnes came to the foot of my bed. "She doesn't look good, does she? I try to encourage her all I can, but sometimes I feel as though she doesn't hear me. She's not fighting for her life. She's giving up, if you know what I mean. How can you help such a one? I guess you just keep trying." Her voice trailed off as she returned to the rumpled bed.

Agnes fidgeted during Bessie's absence. I heard her

pull open a drawer in the bedside stand. "I wonder if anyone ever reads these Bibles," she said to me.

"I don't know."

She said no more. She was making order in the top drawer, arranging the Kleenex, the massage lotion, the folder of hospital information, and the Gideon Bible.

The walkers returned. I sighed with relief for Bessie as she was given her chair once more and the blanket for her knees. Agnes collected her purse, her coat, and a hand-crocheted cap. "I'm going now," she said, kissing Bessie on the forehead, but she was back in minutes. She had seen the cart of midday trays. "Be sure to eat everything on your tray, Bessie," she ordered. "You must eat to get your strength back. Remember, Herman will be here to see you tomorrow morning, and I'll be back as soon as I can, too. Be sure to eat good."

Bessie smiled, making no promises. For my part, I was hungry and ate well. I turned to comment on how good the food was when I saw that Bessie's plate was untouched. She drank a little milk through a straw.

"I have some medicine for you, Mrs. Bailey." The nurse with the medication tray had suddenly invaded. "I'm going to pour this into your orange juice. You must drink it all, Mrs. Bailey. It's on your chart." Bessie complied. Who could resist when all these fine arrangements were made for her? She drank the juice, the whole cup at once.

Bessie's dinner remained in front of her for what seemed like hours. I had long finished my food and had pushed my table aside. I walked around. I went to the bathroom. I was tempted to move Bessie's table too, but I thought it best not to interfere. Besides, Bessie appeared to be asleep.

"You haven't touched your food." It was the red-haired nurse who had entered again. "That nice piece of meat all cut up for you."

After an awkward pause, the trays were taken out the door. The nurse returned, began to move Bessie to her chair, and smoothed the bed. Bessie may rest at last!

"Oh, here come your doctors, Mrs. Bailey," said the nurse, dropping everything and standing at attention.

Three men entered. Two moved briskly forward, stopping at Bessie's chair. The younger one wore a brown jacket with leather patches on the elbows. The older one was bald; a black tie hung from his neck. The doctor who lingered behind was young and immaculately groomed. He was there to observe and listen.

"How are you this evening, Mrs. Bailey?" The bald one spoke. His voice was high-pitched, with a slight English accent. He bent over Bessie and peered into her face.

Bessie opened her eyes. They were keen. She recognized these men and had much she wanted to ask them. They must not get away before she could formulate her question.

"You're looking better," said the one with the leather patches. His voice was amiable and unrushed. He knew how to talk to old ladies. "Maybe we'll have you home for Thanksgiving."

Bessie struggled against the small talk. She spoke to the older man. "Must I take the orange medicine, Doctor? It upsets my stomach."

"You're nauseated?" The high-pitched voice was tender. "You shouldn't be." He summoned the nurse; together they examined Bessie's chart. Another medication might suit her better. He would try. Did she sleep well? That was good.

Bessie smiled, genuinely reassured. I was satisfied that she hadn't given up as Agnes had feared. The three doctors disappeared as quickly as they had come.

The next morning—Sunday—Bessie's brother, Herman, arrived carrying a department store shopping bag. Bessie was sitting in her chair beside the window.

"Shall I close the blind? The sun is awfully bright," Herman began.

"No, no . . . it feels warm," was Bessie's quick response. She was fully awake.

"Food not tasting good yet?" he asked as he put down the parcel. He removed his jacket and cap. He was wearing the olive-drab shirt and pants of a working man.

"Not yet." She didn't want to talk about the untouched breakfast tray. "What are you bringing me now?" She was considerably more alert this morning.

"Fur hats from Dayton's," said Herman proudly. "They're from the money Jennie sent you for a gift—something you can really use. Only Agnes wasn't sure which kind you'd like best, with or without the ear flaps."

Bessie laid one on her lap and tried the one with the flaps on her head. Herman was quick to notice her fascination; it was a welcome response.

"It looks real nice," he said. "Even a rabbit wouldn't know it from real fur." He'd made her laugh. In a little while, he left and she drifted off to sleep.

Agnes bustled in before Bessie woke. She had gotten up early, she said. Sunday was the only day she had to clean her house. She began straightening the room around Bessie as though she were still in the process of cleaning. Bessie awoke.

"Oh, good, you're awake," Agnes said, taking Bessie's comb out of the drawer. "Several people told me they plan to see you today. Let's fix your hair." Agnes raised the mirror set in Bessie's table. Bessie looked into it blankly, as though her face were not reflected there.

"Let's give you an upsweep," Agnes continued. Yesterday Agnes had told me she tried hard. She was trying now.

Bessie finally responded by bending forward and holding her head erect. She wasn't going to be difficult; Agnes was too kind. The snowy wisps were drawn up from Bessie's neck and rolled over a pin. She was getting a new look, the about-town look, the nape of the neck curved like a question mark.

"You're ready for your company, Bessie dear," said Agnes, removing the loose hairs from the comb. She stepped in front of Bessie and tilted her head. "You look wonderful."

Throughout the day between visits with Walt, Steve, and friends from St. Charles, I learned more about Bessie through the people who came to see her.

"You were a good teacher, Bessie," said a stout woman with glasses perched on the wings of her nose. "So many people have said so since you retired. Just the other day, at the shopping center, I ran into Evelyn Price, who said you were the best teacher she'd ever had. Evelyn Price—used to be Evelyn Giles—she married Ronald Price's boy and went on to business college . . . "

"Yes, I remember Evelyn." Bessie's eyes were bright with remembrance as she smiled at her friend. "I enjoyed teaching very much."

That was it! I felt akin. There was something special

about her—that distinctive grace. She had a singular patience that accepted all who had not come to understand the meaning of her illness—family and friends who went on hoping she'd get well, and doctors and nurses who knew she wouldn't—but failed to see the spiritual well-being beneath the disease. Enlightenment stirred in her that the rest of us glimpsed but darkly, if at all. None who had so competently entered this room was her equal; she was a standard against which all might be measured.

Most of us on the fifth floor dreaded the night. Discomfort intensified as we faced that long span of time. Sleep induced by drugs was unnatural, stripped of healthy dreams. And one would wake up too soon, wondering if another hypo would be necessary.

At the end of this busy Sunday, Bessie and I tried to sleep. My mind was like a traffic jam, full of images left from the long day and surgery days before, and what it might mean for my future. Few of us are optimistic while awake at night. In a day, or possibly two, Walt would take me home, and the nightmare would be over, with just a part of rib left behind. Bessie seemed to be resting; all was quiet on her side of the room. With my mind whirling in a hundred directions, I envied her peace.

The bedside clock registered eleven. I considered turning on my reading light, then remembered I didn't have the book I wanted. I thought of the Gideon Bible in the drawer—pages sticking together, crisp and unused, as readily available as toothpaste in every bedside stand throughout the hospital. The benevolent God with limitless power tucked into a drawer—a blasphemy; our faith had not made us whole. I dozed.

In my sleep I vaguely heard coughing, gagging—that awful orange medicine again!

"I'll put on my call light. A nurse will come," I said, wide awake.

"Mine is on too," Bessie managed to say.

We waited. No one came.

"I need the bedpan."

"I'll get it for you." I knew I could make it out of bed to the bathroom and find the pan in its proper slot.

"Thank you so much," she said as I helped her. "But you shouldn't have to do this. I suppose our nurse is busy with someone else. She'll come, I hope. My bed is badly soiled." Since I was up, I went to the door and looked across to the nurses' station. There was a cluster of personnel on the far side of the circle. My voice brought someone running. "Where is your light cord, Mrs. Bailey? We don't know you need us unless you put on your light." The voice was sweet, but the reproach was unmistakable.

"Both our lights have been on a long time. She is on the bedpan now, but her sheets need changing." Resentment welled up in me. Though Bessie was taken care of very efficiently and our room was soon dark and quiet, I still heard those cutting words echoing in the walls.

Morning came.

I went to the bathroom and sat on the toilet seat, staring at our bedpans, wash basins, and sputum dishes stuck in labeled slots in front of me. The new medication hadn't helped Bessie at all. This colossal place with all its elaborate procedures held no relief for Bessie. I flushed the toilet and came out into the open once more.

I stopped at her bed on my way back to my own.

The morning sun shone white out of a crystal blue sky. How fortunate our window faced east.

"Morning is nice here," I heard her say as I was focusing on downtown Rochester, diminutive under the bright sky.

I quickly turned around. "It really is," I said.

Her face had the sun on it as her head rested on the white pillow of her turned-up bed. Her moist eyes held strength. The strange alertness I had seen yesterday was apparent.

"You look well this morning, Bessie," I said with conviction.

"I guess the new medicine was no better than what I had been taking," she said. Strange she would talk about it. "Things don't always work out," her voice trailed. Again her attention was focused outside the window. Anguish had surfaced into the freshness of the morning. She was drawing strength from the sun.

"That's true," I said. "I'm sorry about last night. Things like that shouldn't happen, should they? It's all so confusing. No one really knows anything." I stopped and laced my fingers. "Only God knows."

Her eyes fixed out the window, she seemed not to listen, but my final words—what were they?—brought her back quickly.

"You are right," she said. "Since God knows, why should we worry?"

My nervous fingers became folded hands. She had lifted the old phrase into the sunshine. If I had had pity for her, it was no longer pity but respect and admiration. I had learned that cancer was not merely a piece of bad fortune that left its victim crushed. From now on I sensed she would be my mentor.

My time came to go home to Walt and Steve. Life

would go on, but now I carried in my mind's eye Bessie's face with the sun on it. . . . *When you walk through fire, you shall not be burned, and the flames shall not consume you. For I am the Lord your God.*

The morning paper had been tossed on the couch where I sat. I often browsed through the obituaries, but not today. I didn't want to read Bessie's name. To me she could not be confined to a mere paragraph.

10

June 1981, Vacationing in Colorado

"Snowmass, Colorado, is the site of our AASA (American Association of School Administrators) seminar this spring. It looks like a wonderful spot, even though we can't ski. Want to come along?" Walt shuffled through an envelope of material and handed it to me.

"Colorado, where I've always wanted to go! Of course. I have a clinic appointment June 10, but that can be changed. What are the dates?"

"We're due to arrive on the 21st. We could leave on the 19th, allowing for travel time." We studied an illustrated brochure of the mountainside resort, its rooms, swimming pools, shops and restaurants—all vacation comforts. "As you can see there are slopes with chair lifts," he added, "it's probably lively in the summer, too, with conventions going on."

This is great, I thought. I had lived long enough without seeing mountains—not since Lynden, Washington, where we lived next door to Mount Baker, nor since Marangu where Mount Kilimanjaro offered its immense presence. For me mountains are celestial places of transcendence, symbols of the something more, the mysteriously indifferent, a glimpse of eternal distance—evidence.

I entered the clinic on June 10th with shoulders back and head erect, facing a challenge. These last two years I had approached these clinic appointments with growing anxiety, for tumors and lymph node involvement were occurring on my right side as well. Twice I had undergone deep and painful minor surgery. No one advocated another radical mastectomy, although that might have been the procedure had this been 1957 rather than 1981.

After checking me over on this day, my doctor called in Dr. P., the surgeon who performed major procedures, for consultation. His presence frightened me. He, too, probed deep into my right armpit.

"There is definite involvement here. How far it extends will be determined during surgery." He looked at me although his words were for Dr. H.

Dr. H. spoke directly to me. "We've discovered more involvement in your right axilla and need to schedule surgery. Dr. P. knows what it entails and will be available for us. May we set a time?"

"Does this have to be immediately? I hope to go with my husband to Colorado this month," I replied.

"When do you expect to be back?" asked Dr. H.

"On July 6th, if all goes as planned." I looked at each in turn. Would they consent to a delay? Would it be wise?

"Your tumors have always been slow growing. I think we could let you go without serious risk." He glanced at his colleague who offered no objection. They both consulted the calendar above the desk. Dr. H. pointed to it and said, "How about July 11?" Dr. P. nodded.

"And you?"

"I appreciate your letting me make this trip. I'll be

back and ready by July 11." My smile was genuine. Things were working out after all.

My reprieve offered a new incentive to planning and packing. An enormous trunk held all our camping gear in our maroon Chevrolet Caprice. We were tenters who never considered owning an RV, tenting every chance we got—Wisconsin, northern Minnesota—avoiding motels on long trips. Besides the tent and sleeping bags, we packed a large box of groceries, two stout coolers, a Coleman lantern and stove, kindling to start open fires, as well as clothing and shoes. This time we also took a plastic zipped wardrobe bag of "street" clothes for the seminar along with the usual cut-offs and old shirts.

At 4:00 A.M. on the morning of June 19th, we slipped in and out of the house like thieves in the night, carrying our provisions to the car. As we journeyed we observed the subtle process of dawn. First the stars began to fade, then trees and buildings appeared as silhouettes. Steam rose from creeks and low areas. Soon trees and buildings became more distinct, having features and colors. The moon faded and clouds took on the colors flashed by the sun. Finally the east formed a stage for the bursting forth of the sun. I knew this was yet another new lease on life, the beginning of yet another new day.

We turned south into Iowa. The "tall corn" state was elegant this year, its flat terrain yielding spacious fields of straight corn rows, lush green. June was not yet tassel time.

Late that afternoon we chose our home for the night in Nebraska's Mormon State Park rich in cottonwood trees. The grounds were covered with purple poppies open by day, closed at night. We pitched our tent, named Bemidji, because it was there we had used it for the first time seven years ago. Now it was a routine procedure after so many years. Having seen a swimming area, we changed into suits and went for it. As we came out of the water refreshed and invigorated, an old gentleman in a ranger uniform reproached us. "You shouldn't have gone beyond the ropes, you set a bad example for the children."

Back at camp we built a fire and dug into our provisions. First we'd have happy hour with a cold drink from our cooler and popcorn prepared in the old-fashioned open-fire popper. We then feasted on beet greens from our garden at home, potato salad made earlier for the first night out, and hamburgers grilled in a hand-held rack over the open fire.

Heading west the next morning, we drove into an enormous cloud that resembled a cave door with lightning streaking willy-nilly all around it. As we entered the cave, we were enfolded by murky fluff. It became so dark that cars drove with headlights on, although no one seemed to slow down or hesitate. As for me, I entered *The Wizard of Oz.* Although this was Nebraska rather than Kansas, I expected to go whirling into the sky with Dorothy. Huge drops of rain hit our windshield—we expected to see hail any minute. We came out on the other side of the cave door into blue sky and sunshine.

After leaving Denver, we climbed the mountains into Arapaho National Forest, where we found a beautiful campground beside Clear Creek, a cool mountain stream. But, of course, there was no vacancy—it was Saturday afternoon! However, we returned the next morning to a picnic area close enough to the stream to hear its sound over the traffic and where we splashed our face and hands in its crystal-clear water. What a treat after the shabby private campground of last evening! Walt built a fire, stirred hot-cake batter, and together with bacon and eggs, we dined in mountain splendor! Our drive that day wound through a scenic canyon on the Colorado River. At one point we stopped to cool our feet in the rushing water's edge. We watched a pair of amazingly agile kayakers bounce through the rapids—obviously they could readily right themselves should they overturn. As we approached Snowmass according to the map, we wondered how anything could be built on this bleak and rugged terrain against the mountainside. Finally a sign assured us we were indeed reaching our destination, and in a few minutes, we drove through a gate where a uniformed officer greeted us. "Johnny Denver is here. The place is crowded," he said. "You'll be staying at the Wildwood Motel directly up the mountain. It's the next-to-the-last building; look for Parking Lot 9." Cars were lining up behind us—where had they come from? We had been alone on the road most of the day.

A long way up, to be sure, but what a place! Our spacious room contained every elegant convenience, including a private deck overlooking spectacular views of mountains to the north. Only ten steps from our room, a large swimming pool sparkled under the clear open sky. After a swim and leisurely dressing in street clothes, we strolled the Tower Mall on a terrace just below us where several restaurants offered a wide choice of dinner menus. We chose the Refectory and enjoyed an excellent sirloin steak with salad bar. Before the evening was over, we had found our other Minnesota delegate and his family from Stewartville. We were asleep by ten o'clock in a king-sized bed, neither of us knowing what to do with the third pillow.

Since there would be quiet time for me while Walt attended seminar sessions, I brought my work, a case of books, letters, and journals to research for a novel about Africa. Reading through these materials that first morning to determine characters and plot, I chose to write the story from the point of view of Steve, our eleven-year-old son. This was a very important decision, for the novel came together well from then on.

My writing career began when I retired from teaching at the close of the 1976 school year. My first effort came about from stories I heard during childhood from my father, an aunt, and especially from my grandmother. Characters, plot, and events surfaced from them, and in May 1979 a novel, *Julia's Children*, was finished. I had trouble finding a publisher, and a file of rejections began to bulge. Dealing with discouragement, I followed the advice of other writers I knew: keep writing—begin a new project! I temporarily shelved *Julia's Children* and turned my attention to notes I had on Africa. (*Julia's Children* was self-published in 1987 by Askeladd Press, followed in 1989 by *Fjord Magic, Getting Acquainted with Norway*, nonfiction for young readers.)

Our deck became for me an open door out upon this earth of ours; my time alone was spent there. I became one with these mysterious mountains; their ancient unexplainable presence today would continue for eons. Another chance to see more of them came when one afternoon Walt and I took a side trip after his last session. On our way to Aspen the day before, we had passed a single-lane highway with a sign reading Maroon Creek Road that led to Whitewater National Forest. Now we returned hoping to be brought closer to the snowcapped peaks. After seven miles a large clear lake at the foot of a lofty mountain peak suggested a dark primeval world, by reflection, drawing into its bottomless depth giant trees, the lofty peak, clouds and blue sky. The whole area that June day was covered with lush green vegetation and wildflowers, white, yellow, purple, and red—the Indian paint brush. Trees, mostly aspens, grew on the slopes. The soil was deep maroon, yielding all this wonder; not strange, the names given to these natural wonders were: Maroon Creek, Maroon Lake, and Maroon Bell Peak.

We parked, laced our boots, and set off on a steep rocky trail following signs that promised a waterfall ahead. On our way we discovered additional companion peaks hidden by Maroon Bell until we came this close. We reached the roaring falls, with its rushing stream at the bottom making us thirsty. We drank from cupped hands.

When Walt returned from his final session at noon on June 25th, we went out to lunch, our final meal at Snowmass, and our last time to dress in tailored white shorts. Our next lodging would be the tent; we had packed and were ready and eager to be off.

We bought groceries at Snowmass Village, then headed south toward McClure Pass. The purple peaks appeared in surprising perspectives with each curve of the rolling highway.

We were looking for a campsite, too, as we viewed all this splendor. We evidently missed one that we had spotted on the map, but we found another after the steep climb to the top of the pass, a forest campground only half full of tenters. We nestled our tent among a cluster of pine trees.

"Elk hunters must have used this site," said Walt as we looked over our site. "See that pole fastened between two trees to hang the carcass." We paused a moment, letting our imagination take on a scenario, then turned our attention to the trail to the creek, our source of water.

As I followed Walt carefully down the steep pathway to the river, I stopped short at the sight of a western tanager perched on a twig close to the water, ignoring us. Although not as rare in mountain forests as our scarlet tanager is in Minnesota and Wisconsin, it was a special moment for me to see this colorful bird: brilliant red head, yellow breast, and black wings.

That evening we baked foil-wrapped potatoes in campfire coals, tossed a big salad, trimmed steaks for broiling, and enjoyed popcorn with beer.

It would be a chilly night here on McClure Pass, so we dressed in flannel pajamas, zipped shut the door and windows of Bemidji, and snuggled into warm sleeping bags. Before falling asleep, I delighted again recalling the western tanager as well as other birds I had seen along the way: meadowlarks at a rest stop in Iowa, a western bluebird on my walks at Snowmass, the gregarious stellar jays, blackbirds with yellow heads, and finally the tiny pine warbler, teasing me with his song, but always hidden from view. As a birdwatcher of sorts, I felt rewarded. A deep sigh, and I was asleep.

The next morning, we entered a flat, dry valley where irrigation sustained cherry orchards loaded with luscious fruit. While filling our canteen with cold water at a rest stop, we found cherries put out for sampling. A crude sign invited us to stop at L. farm.

Climbing switchbacks, we caught glimpses of Ouray, the Switzerland of America, nestled among mountains on all sides, then descended into the historic town of Silverton. We stopped at an antique shop called "Patent Medicines and Sundries," a true reminder of the Old West.

Safari Campground in Durango became our home base for two days; a busload of noisy teenagers from Los Angeles occupied several sites around us. No trees! We had been looking for a forest campground without luck. We made do, however. We faced Bemidji toward a hedge at the far end of the grounds flanking a small creek, giving ourselves privacy. "It would be fun to take the old narrow gauge railroad from Durango to Silverton, don't you think?" suggested Walt the next morning while studying brochures. "We don't have to make reservations, since it says here there may be cancellations."

I cheerfully agreed and the next morning we climbed aboard an 1882-vintage train, hissing steam under its wheels and blowing a steam whistle that echoed among the mountains. We chugged along following the Animas River through the San Juan National Forest where wild roses flourished in the meadows and road beds. We saw old mine sites and abandoned cabins. We stopped several times to take on water, each time sparking the haunting whistle. Once we let off a small group of backpackers. We stepped on the platform at Silverton at noon amid the billows of noisy steam hissing beneath us. After lunching in a Mexican restaurant and looking in on several antique shops, all of us returned to Durango along the same narrow gauge route. I came away convinced that there is no better way to get the feel of the heights and depths of the Rocky Mountains than to be taken by train across trestles and through tunnels. It was already six o'clock when we stopped at Safeway for our dinner ingredients, but since the days were long, we had all the time in the world. It would be chow mein prepared in the hanging kettle this evening made with fresh pork steak. We talked about tomorrow's venture, climbing into the cave dwellings of Mesa Verde.

We started out early in order to enjoy the brilliant red colors created by the rising sun. After a half-hour drive, we entered Mesa Verde National Park and stood in awe before ancient dwellings of the Anasazi Indians, including Cliff Palace, a city of gold, taking on fresh luster from the morning sun, defying history's heavy hand.

According to our guidebook, these dwellings high on the cliff's face sheltered a community seven hundred years ago, long before white men set foot in North America. Due to several years of drought, the homes were abandoned after a hundred years or more. In 1880, six hundred years later, they were discovered by two cowboys looking for lost cattle. According to their own account, these two Weatherill brothers came upon the site in winter and stopped in the morning light, as we had, sitting on their horses, staring at the magnificent city through snowy leafless trees.

At Cliff Palace we climbed a narrow stone walkway leading to the cliff dwellings and saw unmistakable rooms on several stories. Through one square opening, we saw designs etched on the opposite wall. What must have been an open courtyard contained several round silo-like holes called kivas, sacred rooms of the ancients, where they contacted their spirits. Once they were covered, only a ladder leading to the courtyard, where ceremonial dances were held on feast days and work detail on normal days. I felt a strange affinity toward these ancients as we walked around their homes. "Distance of time, embrace us, memory is not big enough to sustain us all." I was adding another line to Peter Schieber's poem (see end of chapter 3).

Not until we had experienced Balcony House was our perspective complete. Its hazardous location demanded the help of a guide, who led us down 150 steps to a wide balcony with a breathtaking view. From there we climbed a forty-foot rope ladder and came to a tunnel barely wide enough for average shoulders. Finally we crossed a ten-foot ridge-walk holding onto a chain. I tried to imagine how it would be to live in an upright world climbing either up or down. I watched crows swooping to and fro; this was a place for wings. Although Walt, who is afraid of heights, swore he would never do this again, we were proud of our courage.

Our next stop was in New Mexico. We visited an active pueblo near Taos where the descendants of Mesa Verde's cliff dwellers now live. It is a village of adobe houses attached to one another two to three stories high, with no running water or electricity. Oddly enough it resembled what we had seen the day before. We bought bread baked in a round-dome outdoor oven called a horno and a wool rug from one of the village weavers. Modern-day Indians in New Mexico conduct a lively tourist trade.

Our route home took us north through eastern Colorado, Wyoming, then to South Dakota's Black Hills. It was raining when we arrived, so we stayed in a motel and set out early in the morning through Wind

Cave State Park, the sky totally blue after rain and the meadow totally green. A buffalo stood like a statue at a crossroad. We were sure he was just another spectacular sign. Not until he lifted his tail against the flies and twisted his mouth around his cud did we decide he was real. Weren't we sure all the buffalo were dead for all time? Not so. As we wound through a rocky wooded area coming to an open meadow, we came across a herd of two hundred or more, docile as the loner we had just seen. We stopped. Some of the buffalo were asleep, others slowly rising and muttering deep sounds. Some bulls were snorting. Although lost to history, these creatures were here for us to see. "Distance of time, embrace all."

As I crawled into my sleeping bag on our last night, I recalled the face of the Taos Indian woman who sold me the round loaf of bread. We smiled. She knew nothing about me except I was a tourist, and I knew little about her except that she handmade this lovely bread. I knew I would like her if I had the opportunity.

Suddenly I remembered what I would face coming home. Strange, I hadn't thought about it until now, the function of my unconscious? Anxiety? I would hold it at bay until July 11th. I have been alive to see Colorado's mountains, Mesa Verde's cliff dwellings, to live outdoors with trees, birds, clouds and wind, to grasp at transcendence, to contemplate distance's embrace, and to rejoice as a child of creation.

11

July 1981, Breast Implant Not an Option

When I opened my eyes after surgery, I was in my hospital room. There was the television set hanging on the wall in front of me. There was Walt sitting in the big leather chair. I expected to wake in the recovery room as I had all other times.

"So close to noon, we were told to bring her directly here," I heard an orderly say to a nurse.

"Her doctors are coming," she replied. "I hope she'll be awake."

The next time I opened my eyes, three men stood at my bedside, only one wearing a white coat. I felt awkward the way they stared at me. *Do they know I read Tolstoy and write poetry? That I am me?* Turning my head I saw that Walt had left the chair and was coming closer. My eyes closed again; I was not yet capable of sustaining consciousness.

"Perhaps it's a little early for her," the doctor in the white coat was saying to Walt, "but all three of us happened to be here just now and have matters to discuss with her."

I woke quickly hearing this and mustered enough alertness to greet them. Walt took my hand.

"We are recommending a course of radiation for

you," Dr. P. began. "This is Dr. S.," indicating the bearded one, "who will arrange for you to see him after you leave the hospital."

"Radiation?"

"We want to tell you why," continued Dr. P. "We need to treat tumors that were too close to the main artery and nerve to successfully remove during this surgery."

"You mean something is still there?" I tried raising myself off the pillow. I was too sedated.

"We are quite confident radiation will take care of it, but it must begin at the proper time." Who said this I couldn't tell.

"I'll be looking for you one of these days," said the bearded one, touching my shoulder, as the other two moved toward the door.

Just as they were leaving a violent surge of pain ran through my right shoulder. I panicked. Something was left, they said. "I'm dying!" I called out to Walt, who still held my hand. "Just now I have unbearable pain!"

"I'll call a nurse," Walt tried to let go my hand.

"No, no, you mustn't leave me!"

A nurse entered abruptly. "I have a shot for pain," she said. "I had to wait until your doctors left. There, now. I'm sorry you had to wait for this one."

Oblivion returned. I vaguely knew Walt would be in the big leather chair.

Just as day was breaking, Jesus stood on the beach; yet the disciples (out in their fishing boat) did not know it was Jesus . . . Through the mist on the lake, I saw Him. He was standing beside my bed looking down at me. I knew Him by the kindness in His eyes.

"Peace? I didn't quite hear You."

"You are awake?"

I focused my eyes and saw it was Pastor T. "I'm sorry. I think I was dreaming. I thought you were . . . Him." Would he be embarrassed knowing I had mistaken him for Our Lord? He simply smiled, but was in no hurry to speak.

Awake now, I studied our new pastor. I had been on the committee that called him. His gentle and unassuming presence totally surprised me. Had he just now called out to his disciples? How had I linked him with the man on the beach? He was not tall or robust, had slightly stooped shoulders, and wore a shirt open at the neck. He was simply a friendly young man here to greet me.

"I only came to say hi," he said as I placed my hand in his. "I'll come another day, soon."

"So glad you came. Don't hurry away," I said, feeling uneasy. There seemed to be a rush of people in and out of the room, very little recognition.

Walt stood beside us now. "Thanks for coming," he said to Pastor T. "Given time, she'll be on the mend."

"I'm sure." The pastor smiled again. "Prayers are being said for you. Good-bye," he said, pressing my hand before dropping it. Peace like a wave came over me. Walt walked with him to the door.

Returning, he said, "It's a bit early for you to have company. You'd better take it easy."

"I'm happy he came. What a nice person!"

"I'll bet you'll sleep again. May I go out for a bite to eat?"

"Do. I'll be all right."

It was early evening when I awoke; I had slept through the dinner hour. I was not particularly hungry.

I was surprised at the lapse of time. I suddenly noticed I had a roommate as the curtain between our beds fluttered, and I heard voices.

"I'm going home tomorrow as soon as the doctor gets here to discharge me," said the first voice.

"You'll be a model as ample as a Barbie Doll," said a male voice, laughing at his own remark.

A silicon-gel implant is what they were talking about, and it had happened to her. It had never occurred to me to have such a procedure; it somehow seemed frivolous. Besides, I lived with a prosthesis as easily as wearing a bra, or shoes, for that matter. The plastic surgeon who excised all my nodules and did extensive grafting on my chest wall was skillful at breast implants and undoubtedly did my neighbor's, but for me the subject never came up. If nodules kept recurring under an implant, what then? It was understandable that it was never brought up. *My husband accepts me as I am,* I thought, *and that's all that matters.*

After the man left, she drew back the curtain slightly and said, "Mind? I'm so excited about going home tomorrow, I can't sit still."

"Not at all! I am wide awake. Not going home tomorrow, I'm afraid, not until I shed these IV tubes."

She opened the curtains all the way and came closer. She had the window side of the room, and I had the door. "What did they do to you? Most patients in this section of the hospital are women with cancer."

"I had a mastectomy twenty-four years ago. My battle is recurring malignant nodules in the area of the original scar. This time these nodules were found on the other side, under my arm, and a probe was made, some tumors left behind for radiation to take care of.

Had this been 1957 instead of 1981, they would have taken my right breast also. That procedure is less frequent these days."

"Twenty-four years! You're a survivor! You must be one of those positive thinkers, mind over body. I've heard positive thinking is a big factor."

"Others have told me that, but I'm not bragging." I laughed a little. "Can you crank me up a little so I can see you better? Thanks. Now what about you?"

She moved to the other side of my bed. "I had a mastectomy two years ago. It was a terrible shock; I was only thirty-six years old!"

"I know what you mean."

She stood there, a beautiful young woman in her red velour robe. Her honey-colored hair was brushed in place, hardly belonging to one who had been in a hospital bed. She had an easy smile, engaging eyes. "Now you've had an implant?"

"How did you guess?" she asked.

"To be honest, I overheard." I pushed my feet against the sheets to keep from sliding. "Besides, I can tell you're happy about something."

"You bet. You want to see?" Without waiting for an answer, she spread the front of her robe. "Not bad, is it? The stitches will be gone in another ten days."

"Dr. W. must have done your surgery—beautiful job."

"Why? Do you know him?"

"He has been treating me for years, removing malignant nodules from my left chest wall and grafting where skin becomes tight and thin. They don't come any nicer than he. His smile is enough to reassure his patients, no matter what he plans to do to them."

"You aren't kidding." She began moving to her side

of the room. "I better let you rest. I've tired you out with my chatter. Do you want your bed lowered?"

"No, I'm fine. I'm waiting for my husband. He'll be here before bedtime." And sure enough, I glanced toward the door and there he stood holding a large, gift-wrapped parcel with a huge blue bow.

"May I come in?"

"You sure may! Say hi to my roommate."

He greeted her, then placed the parcel on the bed. "I'll bet you thought I'd never come back. I've been shopping."

"So I see. Where did you go?"

"Masseys—nothing but the best."

"Masseys?"

"To tell the truth, yesterday morning one of your fellow teachers handed me an envelope. 'Get her something she can use right away,' so I went to Masseys. Now you will see what I got!"

"They must have grown tired of sending me flowers and plants," I said as I removed the huge bow, the decorative paper, and lifted the lid. Rustling the white tissue paper, I lifted a flowered garment. "A housecoat! How beautiful. You don't mean to tell me you picked it out?"

"I had help. The clerks there like to wait on men who are buying gifts for their wives. The attention was kind of nice."

I gave him an understanding smile. "Tomorrow I'll wear it. Then I hope to be up and around."

Walt left when a nurse came to prepare us for the night.

Dr. W. arrived just as our breakfast trays were carried out. I would have missed him if I hadn't heard him talking to my roommate behind the curtain. "There is no reason to stay here any longer, young lady. You're going home," he announced. I knew just how he was smiling at her.

"I am so pleased, Doctor. My whole life has changed!"

"That's how we want you to feel. Good-bye, and have a safe trip home."

Dr. W. turned and stopped at my bedside. "Mrs. Gilseth, here again?" He meant this as a greeting. "I know—those nodules under your right arm. I'll see your report."

"You did great work for my roommate—she's so happy."

"Wish we could do the same for you." He patted my cheek with the back of his hand. "But you know why, don't you?"

"You've given me years to live, Dr. W., excising all my nodules. I am more grateful to you than I can say."

"Thanks for that," he said, about to go his way, "You're a friend of long standing." We both smiled as he left.

A nurse came after my midday nap. "I'm getting you up for a walk. You did fine this morning." She brought my new housecoat from the closet. "You're really quite elegant, I'd say," she continued as she helped me into it. The IV bag dangling from its stand had to go with us as together we went into the hall. "Brand new? A gift, I'll bet. Our hospital gowns don't do much for patient morale." On our return we passed a little cove with a table, a lamp, and two comfortable chairs. I made a mental note; I'd be back. "You're doing great. Next time we'll let you do it alone," she said as we entered the door. She left me sitting in my chair.

He was in the room before I noticed him. "You're sitting up! I don't have to ask how you are, I can see how well you're doing." It was Pastor T., who'd said he would return another day.

"I'm so happy to see you. Grab a chair from the other side of the curtain. No one is there at the moment."

Before he went for the chair, he went to my bedside stand where lay a copy of *Prayers of Kierkegaard.* "This yours? You read Kierkegaard?" He held up the little volume. "Difficult stuff, isn't it?"

I felt something interesting coming on. "On second thought, let's go to the little cove across the hall from here. The chairs are better." I began to move, carefully rolling my IV with me. Pastor T., carrying the book, took my arm as we went through the door.

"I can't say I always know what I am reading," I began as we sat across from each other at the little table, "but I always find some wonderful kernels, gems, that keep me going."

"I'm learning more about you," he said, smiling, "What people read says a lot about them."

"His philosophical discourses are pretty much beyond me. I stick with his religious writings. *Fear and Trembling* got me started when I was in a period of depression. It helped me a great deal."

"Many seminary students give up on Kierkegaard; you know that, don't you?"

"But not you?"

"By no means. I think he says it all."

"Good! Then I know something about you, too." A smile of kinship broke between us.

"Would you like me to read you one of these?" he

said, turning pages in the book he had not yet laid down.

"Before surgery I read number 9 on page 14. I would love to hear it."

> "Thou who has first loved us, O God, alas! We speak of it in terms of history as if Thou hast only loved us first but a single time, rather than without ceasing Thou hast loved us first many times and everyday and our whole life through. . . . And yet we always speak ungratefully as if Thou hast loved us first only once."

The hospital surroundings, its impersonal sights and sounds and smells, disappeared as we sat together for this moment of reading. After visiting pleasantly about St. Charles—new to him—we returned to my room, I to my chair. He left as quietly as he had come.

Walt arrived soon after with a plant of yellow mums, this time from my circle of churchwomen. Two other floral arrangements had arrived from friends yesterday; there was hardly room for all of them.

"Nice to find you sitting up and wearing the gown. It looks great on you!" Walt found room for the plant on a shelf near the TV. "I met Pastor T. in the hall. He was impressed with the way you're recovering."

After Walt left, a nurse returned me to my bed. "Enough for one day," she said, "In another hour, your supper tray will arrive. Rest if you can."

There were voices at my door. An escort brought in a woman, a man, and a boy, perhaps twelve or fourteen. As the man asked questions of the escort, I quickly recognized by his accent that they had just arrived from a foreign country. After the escort left, they spoke in what I recognized as German, but I could not understand them. Although they were pleased with the room, I sensed that they were sober and anxious. The man and the boy left as a nurse came to do preliminary preps. The woman was as articulate in English as her husband, answering questions put to her.

The supper trays arrived and we were propped up with our adjustable tables in front of us.

"Do you want your curtain open or closed?" asked the aide before she left.

"I prefer it open," I replied, not sure of my roommate's preference. It was hastily pushed aside.

We looked at each other. I felt I should speak first. "It's no fun to be put to bed at this time of day when there is seemingly no need."

"It's a bit strange, but I don't mind. My name is Elizabeth Hofter. I come from the Federal Republic of Germany. We arrived yesterday." She seemed eager to talk, even though it meant using her second language. "I need to have my breast taken off, but at home I had to wait so long to have it done. Here I was taken right in."

We uncovered the serving dishes on our trays—a piece of swiss steak with mashed potatoes and gravy, red Jell-O and a cup of sherbet for dessert. "You'd better eat everything. You won't get any breakfast in the morning." I wondered about her reaction to the food before her.

"What a large piece of meat, enough for two people. Everything is quite elegant here." She began to eat with her fork in her left hand.

She listened intently as I introduced myself and related to her my prognosis. She was not afraid to ask me to repeat if she didn't understand. When I stopped, she said, "They have done wonders for you in this place, I can see. I have every reason to hope things will go well for me, too."

Her husband and son returned while we were finishing our sherbet. She introduced them and they nodded toward me, bowing from the waist. Although formal, the greeting was warm; the teenager well-mannered. They had followed a tour guide book sightseeing around the city, and another day planned to rent a car.

"Here are our other two sons," she said reaching for a picture she had already placed on her bedside stand. "We left them with my parents. Eugene wanted to come. We thought he would learn much making the trip with us." The boy smiled at his mother as she looked at him. "And it's nice to have the two of them with me now."

I was grateful to this woman. I felt unexpectedly close to her as she spoke of her family. She had brought hope, another dimension into this room. I knew she was vulnerable; I would pray for her.

The next morning after eating the breakfast I couldn't share with her, the cart from surgery arrived. Her husband and son were there as she received her Demerol shot, the initial sedation, and they watched her being lifted onto the cart and covered with a flannel blanket. I knew what the journey to the operating theater was like; it was traumatic in spite of Demerol. I looked at the husband and saw Walt's anxious face, at the son and saw Steve's troubled eyes. I remembered years ago how I followed my father on his journey; he lay paler than I had ever seen him and, although he seemed asleep, there was tumult beneath his lids.

"Good luck." I waved as she rolled by, followed by

her husband and son. It was frivolous to say, but common usage around here to lighten the atmosphere.

Two days later, as I was ready to leave the hospital, I felt reluctant to let go this good friend. I had answered many of her questions asked me as we visited. Where could she get a prosthesis like the one I had? I wrote down the name of the store that carried them and encouraged her to buy a swimsuit and put a pocket in it for her form. "Your life need not change; your maturity will help a lot," I said. We parted, promising to keep in touch, at least a card at Christmas.

At the time scheduled for me, I went to see Dr. S. in the Currie Pavilion where radiation patients are treated. I scarcely remembered him except for his beard and his matter-of-fact demeanor. He marked me with an indelible ink spot, which would last the entire three weeks of treatment, indicating where the radiation was to penetrate. I was to come in every day except Saturdays and Sundays. I had a question for him before he left to see another patient. "My family has a ten-day canoe trip planned for the second week in August. My treatments will not be completed by then, I know, but I would like to go with them then."

"Canoeing?" He gave me a dubious look. I was sure he would say the risk of being in the sun would be too great. "It's an unusual request, I must say. Canoeing where?"

"On the St. Croix," I replied, puzzled at the look on his face.

"If you keep yourself carefully covered, especially your shoulders, I guess we can risk it."

An unexpected surprise. "I'll live by the rules. Thank you, Doctor."

12

The 1980s, Volunteering in the Third World

"Your chest x-ray should be up from the lab by now. I'm going to check on it and will be back in a minute," said Dr. H. "You may get dressed." He was apparently finished with me, but not quite.

It was a beautiful day in June 1984, and I was in a sterile, tiny room on the twelfth floor of the Mayo Clinic having a routine check-up. After dressing I stood at the window and gazed out at the city of Rochester and the countryside beyond, anxious to get out into this summer day.

Nothing major had developed following two courses of radiation during the fall of 1981. I was given a new drug called tamoxifen and told that in a case such as mine we could expect favorable results. Three years later, however, in February and March of this year, nodules again appeared on my chest wall, at which time Dr. W., my plastic surgeon, removed them. These new incisions were slow to heal, and there was slight but troublesome drainage. My regular check-ups became more frequent, as often as every other month. Dr. H. found nothing threatening today. "Given time, those abrasions will heal," he said, and I had no reason not to believe him.

I left the window and sat on the stiff leather couch. He seemed to be taking a while. Then the door opened abruptly. He brought an x-ray film with him, which was unusual, and tucked it in a holder above the desk. Something was wrong.

"You have two small tumors on your lungs." He looked at me as a father who hoped to drive home the seriousness of what he was saying. *Me? Is that really my x-ray film? Might it not belong to someone else?* I wasn't ready to claim it. Should I stand up as he was pointing out the awful truth to me? I remained seated. I saw as much as I could be expected to understand.

"So what now?" I began sinking inside as he looked toward me.

"There are a number of options." Now he sounded less threatening. "Tamoxifen worked well for you for a time; I believe you respond to hormones better than most. But obviously it is not working for you now, so stop those pills right away."

This was step one. *Something can be done about it,* I thought.

"I'm going to prescribe another hormone, halotestin. Since it is a male hormone, you may see some side effects such as excessive facial hair and a lowering pitch to your voice—masculine characteristics—nothing major."

"This is not chemotherapy, then?" I said, which was my greatest dread.

"No, hormone therapy is much easier to take. We'll try it for a while." He began writing on a pad of prescription blanks. "Come back in another two months and we'll see how this is working." He tore off the sheet and handed it to me. I wanted to ask questions but couldn't find words. He held the door open for me and lay a reassuring hand on my shoulder as we parted in the corridor. I tried to smile.

"It's not good news, Walt. It's in my lungs." He stirred in the waiting room chair and laid the newspaper aside. He may not have heard me I spoke so softly. "It's not good news," I repeated as he rose.

"I heard." He took my arm. "Let's go."

"This is liable to be it, Walt."

"This has been a long wait. What do you say we go to Great China for their noon buffet? I'm sure you are as hungry as I am."

He walked me to the elevator. I began to calm down with him at my side. Was anything so terribly wrong? We were going out to eat.

I deliberately chose to delight in the beautiful summer days that followed. I walked around the garden frequently, examining the flourishing tomato, cabbage, and pepper plants. The cucumbers were throwing out vines not to mention the prolific zucchini.

At an outdoor family barbecue in our backyard one Sunday afternoon, it occurred to me that none of my extended family knew about my current state of health. Bring up such a subject? I couldn't. Walt wasn't saying anything either; perhaps he thought it was none of their business. I would, however, tell our son Steve.

Inconspicuously I drew him and Walt with me into our little A-frame guest house among the trees at the edge of the yard. We sat on twin beds across from one another as I explained what my x-ray had revealed. "I thought you should know, Steve, what the score is with your mother." It was out at last.

"I always said you would live to a ripe old age, and I say it again." Like his father, Steve was sensitive and caring but didn't try to express his feelings in words. I could have predicted he would make light of it.

I rose as a signal they could leave. "That's it, guys. Let's join the others."

Soon I was living with this new development as readily as before. When a flutter of panic came, I remembered that another appointment was coming up; things were being dealt with. *They that trust in the Lord shall renew their strength . . .* I shared my thoughts and feelings with Pastor T. on his frequent visits to the house to exchange *The Christian Century* for *Christianity and Crisis*, along with books. We could talk to one another, he and I, and I shared my concerns without fear.

Excitement stirred one day when Walt returned from Mankato, where he had delivered a year's supply of eyeglasses collected by our small town's Lions Club. I had no sooner gone out to meet him than he called out, "How would you like to go to Mexico?"

"I'm ready to go almost anywhere. Mexico, you say?"

"A team of optometrists belonging to a group called VOSH (Volunteer Optometrists in the Service of Humanity) plan to travel to Parral, Mexico, this coming February to distribute free glasses. They need helpers to work in their clinic. It's not so easy to find these people since each would have to pay his own way."

"For how long?" I asked.

"The clinic lasts five days plus travel time, with some interesting stops if we want to make them—I'd guess two weeks at the most."

We discussed this unexpected possibility on comfortable chairs in the backyard. We would have to make periodic trips to Mankato to help prepare the glasses for distribution. They had to be sanitized in detergent, dried, read for their prescription, labelled, put in plastic bags, sorted, and finally packed in boxes according to their prescription. At least four thousand pairs of glasses would be needed to service a five-day clinic. They would be sent ahead to be on hand for the team when they arrived.

I listened as Walt continued. "February is a long way off, I know, but we could tentatively sign on and go through the motions." We both knew a lot could happen between now and then, and silently we acknowledged the fact.

"Coming just now, this is a wonderful opportunity. I'm all for it," I said.

The draining incisions became more troublesome when I first began taking the new pills. After a few days, however, I noticed that healing was indeed taking place until finally there was a clean scar. In August I returned to Dr. H. who was pleased with my progress.

"Your changed medication certainly enhanced the healing of those stubborn incisions. I don't find any nodules, so I think we can assume that this hormone is working for you. You may get dressed, I'll check your x-ray." He was out the door. I was scarcely dressed when he returned. "One of the tumors we saw last time is gone, the other is barely visible. We're definitely on the right track. You continue to amaze me. How long has it been now? Twenty-seven years, I believe."

"I'm very grateful—you have taken good care of me," I said.

"I think the 'Man Upstairs' has something to do with it," he said as he wrote out my prescription. This statement struck me as flippant small talk, but no matter, it was true. "Take only one a day from now on."

I had yet another reprieve—I left with a light heart. The door was open for a new experience. On February 14, 1985, we were on our way to Mexico with the VOSH team prepared to hold clinics in two cities, Camargo and Parral. Maps give sterile impressions of a place; only when we find ourselves in the sky above a country and landing in a city or traveling down a dusty road do we open our eyes to what is real.

Landing in El Paso, Texas, we were met and helped through customs by a delegation of Lions from Camargo, ninety miles away. We waited for what seemed like hours in an old school bus while our passage was being authorized before crossing the border into Juarez, Mexico. We hadn't eaten since breakfast on the early morning flight to Denver and were famished.

As the smelly old bus groaned along, the contrast between the two border cities was startling. El Paso was a sophisticated city nurtured by a U.S. Texas economy while Juarez stood in the rubble. Other signs that we were in Mexico were the colorful tile even on crumbling walls, people out on the streets—many women and children—and young people selling flowers at intersections. Occasionally a donkey cart with a family in it, a part of the bleak, rocky terrain. There may have been grassy lawns behind courtyard walls, traditional Mexican style. We left the bus in Juarez and boarded a small aircraft, destination Chihuahua, and landed on a long, bumpy runway, uneven with rocks and burned grass.

Without benefit of food, the most tiring of all this day was the three-hour bus ride out of Chihuahua through clay and rock desolation to Camargo, the first city where half of our people were prepared to set up a clinic. We saw the sun go down, a dusky auburn, and daylight slip away. After a dusty detour, we arrived at Camargo's Motel Los Nogales, where a delegation of Lions met us and we were assigned rooms.

What happened next was unbelievable! We were ushered into a large hall where women from the city's Lions Club had spread a long buffet with salads, breads, casseroles, and desserts extending its entire length. Toasts followed the dinner, a series of welcomes and thank-yous carried out with great formality. There was music, too, and we danced until midnight following this exhausting day.

We made three trips to Mexico with VOSH, this one, and two more to Etzatlan, a smaller town, near Guadalahara during February of 1986 and 1988. My medication continued to keep my cancer in remission. I had good reason to stay alive for our involvement with VOSH was yielding surprises and rich rewards. Although the Lions, the towns' elite, were most hospitable, providing housing, meals, and interpreters throughout our stays, getting close to the common folks who formed the long lines waiting for hours to get into our clinics touched me the most. Hope kept them out there—how strong they must be—yet resignation surely went hand in hand with this hope. What if the supply runs out? Then it would be necessary to go back home, nothing changed, but life would go on. One woman in her eighties, totally blind with cataracts, sat in a corner of our waiting area, a little white terrier under her chair. She held him on a rope leash attached to a little red collar. "The dog leads her around the streets," my interpreter explained to me. "We all know her here in our town." Although she had waited with the crowd all afternoon, there was nothing we could do for her. She and her little terrier would continue to cope together.

One day an old farmer who had undoubtedly walked a long way to the city handed me his prescription. He had obtained it from the optometrist and was now about to receive his glasses. I, a supplier, took his prescription and searched to almost no avail until I found a very small pair, undoubtedly made for a woman, that would hardly fit this man. It was worth a try. He was satisfied that he could see well through the lenses, so I took him to the fitters, who dipped bows in hot sand and used small screwdrivers to adjust frames, to see if anything could be done. "How can you expect these to fit this man? We don't give away junk!" The fitter tossed the glasses into the trash bin.

"Sorry" was all I could say. It was late in the day, and I knew there were no more glasses of his prescription. I watched him put on his hat and walk out silently with no change of expression. I was distraught. Why did J.D. have to be so abrupt? Might we not have saved the lenses and looked for another frame? The long clinic hours were taking their toll.

Most people left our clinic happy and expressed their thanks. Women proved they now could thread their needles. A priest could now read prayers during mass; heretofore he had carried out all his masses by heart because he couldn't see to read. "I won't stumble now that I can see," a ninety-four-year-old woman told me through my interpreter. An eight-year-old boy who needed very thick lenses was helped by one of our team members who worked a whole morning putting together a pair by taking lenses out of separate frames incorporating them into a new pair. "It won't work every time, but it's worth a try," he said. Perhaps the most satisfying was to find glasses for children with sight problems. Busloads of them would come to our clinic for screening, and many needed glasses. Walt carried a gross of pencils with him and gave one to each of them, enjoying their smiles of thanks.

There were times when we did not live by the rules. I caught two farmers from the country trading glasses for a look, something they were told not to do, and they came to me and said they saw better in the other's glasses. I read their prescriptions again and assured them a trade would be okay. They both smiled their thanks and went away happy. Another old gentleman told us his wife could see well with the glasses he wore and asked if we had a pair for her. My interpreter and I stowed away a pair for her in his shirt pocket. "Gracias!"

Our large fashionable frames were popular with the women, although they were not in everyone's prescription. The fortunate ones were delighted, which led to others asking, "Don't you have a pair like that for me?" Sunglasses were another prize in short supply and kept only for those who worked in the sun all day. One woman, delighted with her glasses, exclaimed to me, "You will go straight to heaven."

A crisis developed for us at our second clinic: customs demanded exorbitant duty before releasing our glasses. After long deliberation they were finally given over to us at 6:00 P.M. on the third day of our clinic. In the meantime we worked with glasses left in the town from a previous clinic plus what one of our optometrists brought with him, a small fraction of our need. I marveled that we could function at all; it was like the "five loaves and two fishes," seeing the long lines of folks and our meager supply to give away. Soon a skeleton crew resorted to screening and preparing prescriptions for people who would return when the glasses were released. The whole town knew of our predicament, and as we walked the streets, people would give us silent looks of hope and resignation in the same glance.

We made use of our free time the second morning walking to the outskirts of the town to get the feel of how the people lived. Evidently there were no zoning laws; people had their animals with them. We had been hearing roosters crowing and dogs barking every morning; now it was not unusual to see goats and donkeys. A woman was scrubbing clothes on a board in a big tub; the soapy water was dumped in the gutter alongside the road where we walked. Soon a boy of twelve or thirteen began to follow us—not unusual we were told. They were not beggars, simply curious. The boy wanted to practice the little English he knew; we, in turn, practiced a little Spanish.

He led us down a road to a cabinet-making factory. Looking through a small door off the street, we saw ten or more young men, in their twenties, sawing, planing, sanding, and carving. Carefully handcrafted chairs with curved legs and carved backs were coming off their production line while a boombox with loud rock music entertained them. They were proud of their work and were happy to show us around.

Our young friend stayed with the carvers while we continued back toward the city square. The streets of the town were of cobblestone, shiny and clean. The walking area of the square itself was covered with colorful tile; alongside were flowerbeds of blooming roses. Someone was always caring for the square, tending the flowers and sweeping the walkways. Furthermore, in front of each shop surrounding the square, someone was out sweeping. I enjoyed the square for writing my journal in the morning, and we enjoyed it at night when it became lively with gaily dressed young people and mariachi bands. Worshipers filed in and out of the church on Sunday mornings, the most prominent building in the square, which enthroned in bright blue the Blessed Virgin in the high altar. After seeing the excruciating crucifix within its walls, I was troubled, knowing how people who suffer identify with the dying Jesus.

Outside the city of Etzatlan was a colony of several Americans who came to Mexico to spend the winter. They rented space from an American-turned-Mexican who owned a small ranch. While visiting there I met a gentleman who had moved to Mexico seeking help for cancer. His disease was now in remission, and he was ecstatic about the well-being he was experiencing since receiving help here. We compared notes: he was on a female hormone and I on a male. We shook hands on it, wishing each other well.

South of Etzatlan was a mountain on top of which stood a huge cross visible for miles. "Want to go up there?" It was the American-turned-Mexican, who offered to take us in his 1941 vintage, two-ton army jeep he kept alive with Dodge parts. The road was extremely rocky and full of narrow hairpin curves; only those who could hang on tight would survive. The cross was a treacherous hike beyond where we parked; a strong wind made it extremely difficult to reach. At the base of the cross were mysterious-looking worshipers, perhaps monks. From there we were awed by the fantastic view of the city and of the green squares we were told were wheat fields. Etzatlan is a very old city, which once had a thriving silver mine during pre-revolution days. Soon after that it was overmined and became so deep that it filled with water and buried all the equipment.

One day Sarah, one of our young interpreters, suggested we travel to a three-hundred-year-old hacienda. An American from the colony took a group of us in his pickup truck. I rode in the cab while the others had to survive in the back. We drove over what was scarcely a field road, stopping to open and close gates. No one lived there except for one or two hands during harvest. The kitchen was still intact and used occasionally; old fruit trees, grapefruit, lime, tangerine and banana, overran the courtyard; one could have a meal right here. We stepped into the ruins of the hacienda church, the walls still standing after three hundred years. Tall caster bean weeds had taken over the sanctuary. There was no sign of life among the ruins except for birds, a herd of goats, and twenty or more hives of bees. Caught up again in "distance of time," I pictured a day when this place was teeming with a hundred people or more, peasant families working for the landlord under the shadow of the church. Hope must have been alive among them, and resignation.

Upon leaving Etzatlan, we prized the friendship we had made with the people in the home that housed us, Antonia and her daughter, Lucy, a teacher. We exchanged gifts our last evening together and used a Spanish-English dictionary for an hour's conversation.

With my cancer still in remission, another opportunity came for us, in December of 1989, during a VOSH trip to Arusha, Tanzania, Africa, less than a hundred miles from where we had lived four wonderful years thirty years ago. We had never been back. The acute nostalgia I suffered the first years after our return from this assignment had crystallized over these many years into memories of moments, places, and people enriching my joy in them. I was ready to go back for a visit.

We were part of a large, well-organized team from Missouri who were happy to have us as interpreters. Our clinics were set up for us in the surrounding villages by the Rotary Club of Arusha. Though causing hardship, moving each day to a different village was a unique adventure for our entire team. As Walt and I greeted people up and down the waiting line, our teammates began to recognize what we already knew; these were not simply a crowd of black, primitive strangers, but friendly people with big smiles and alert facial expressions. We ran into individuals in the lines who knew of Marangu where we had taught and were delighted to make our acquaintance. One not-so-young recognized me, exclaiming, "You came into our standard-two classroom and taught us a song—I never forgot you—I still sing the song." Since affordable optometric service was extremely scarce in this area, we found many teachers, government workers, and clergy in the line. "Now I can see to read God's Word," an elderly pastor said to me by way of showing gratitude.

During our clinic in the village of Mbuli bordering Maasailand, Emanueli Malisa, our most memorable former student, appeared. Stationed in this village as an education officer, he came to the hospital to see what was going on and discovered us. What a celebration for Walt and me! What an astonishing impression was made on our colleagues with all our exclaiming, hugging, and picture-taking! "These were my tutors," he kept telling everyone as he was being introduced.

Among the nine hundred pairs of glasses distributed that day was one to a young man who required a prescription of 2500, and we had it available! "The highest power I've ever run across among people I have examined anywhere is 1700," examined the optometrist who examined him. "This pair has been riding around with us for a long time." It was hard to assess the astonishment of the young man who received the glasses. He was speechless, he just kept nodding.

After leaving our VOSH mates on their way home, we arrived in Marangu and checked in at the Kibo Hotel where all the climbers of Kilimanjaro stay. When they learned we were not mountain climbers but former teachers at the college who had returned for a visit, we were treated like long-lost friends, first by hotel personnel and soon by people in the streets who greeted us.

Walking about became a social event. "I wasn't born when you were here," one spritely boy exclaimed. "I was just a little child," said another. Suddenly someone recognized us. He had been the school's maintenance man, now retired, and his son had taken his place. "Do you still play the organ?" we asked, remembering how he had not only played, but skillfully repaired faulty organs, while I taught music those years. "My son plays at church now," he responded and quickly continued, "You must come and visit me. You know where I live!" (We did before leaving Marangu.)

Our most delightful discovery was that Apaphra Moshi, one of our students, was now the head of the school. He had studied in the United States, then received his Ph.D. in London, England. The school had grown from one hundred to four hundred students, with a faculty of forty, all Tanzanians. He embraced us as Emanueli had done; it was a celebration! We reminisced about the choir of those days, the work camps in the bush and practice teaching, and we signed two guest books. After introducing us to some of his faculty and giving us tea and "ground nuts" in the dining room, with pride he showed us around the campus, among the buildings we remembered as well as the new buildings. Among them was a science laboratory, a larger library, and a new chapel. I stood in wonder at the landscaping; flowerbeds and blooming trees were more beautiful than I ever remembered them. Early one morning we climbed the open stairs behind the main building to view Mount Kilimanjaro as we used to do. Sunrise yields the best time to catch a total picture, since after that it is usually covered with clouds.

Was our old cook still alive? No one we talked to had heard that he was dead, so we made a trip into the next village where we knew he lived and found an old friend of his, a carpenter who led the way on a two-mile trail past homes under banana trees. We found him among his coffee trees, examining a handful of red beans. He looked up at his guests, then recognized us immediately. "Salaam! So we meet again!" he exclaimed, bringing tears to our eyes.

After he lead us into his house, we reminisced: "Remember the time we served zebra meat to the visiting German bishops?" asked Walt. "They never knew it was the best we could bring in from our hunt." The old gentleman nodded and smiled, looking around at his family who had never heard the story.

"You liked the bread I made," he said finally, pride glistening in his eyes.

Around the corner from the Kibo Hotel stood Nguruma Church, although not as we remembered it. Now it was a beautiful new place of worship, shaped round like a Chagga hut, with space for eight hundred to a thousand people. The bell was still in the tree, requiring an agile boy to climb into it and kick the bell into swinging. We were overwhelmed with the special love we received that Sunday morning, the last day of our stay. In this sanctuary crowded with people, we were invited to stand in the chancel before them with a greeting. In turn a special song was offered us, one we remembered well. Choked with emotion we returned to our pew amid an outburst of clapping. As we filed out singing the last hymn, I was touched by the beauty of this setting out here on the mountain. A bird, perched on the cross atop the church, called out between stanzas. Foliage, flowers, and trees enveloped us. Homes are concealed by them. There is no slaughter of trees.

Throughout the 1980s I experienced a revived solidarity with the human family. Among my American colleagues, I had seen tireless dedication to making life better for those with less, tying fortunes together for the good of all. I had seen people in other lands not different but like myself. Among them I experienced community—belonging. What we had in common was hope, the one essential quality of the human spirit; but, as I came to recognize, it was linked to resignation. What better lesson could there be for one living with cancer?

Epilogue

I saw Steve standing next to Walt as I was rolled into my hospital room after two hours of surgery. They had been waiting patiently. "I brought Steve," said Walt, "I thought you would be glad to see him."

"I am glad. Hi, Steve."

"Hi." He came closer after I had been transferred to my bed. "I hope they didn't treat you too badly."

After keeping me in remission for eight years, the hormone halotestin began to fail me. Early in 1991 nodules were periodically removed over a period of three months. Now five nodules had sprung up simultaneously, needing urgent attention. In addition to the excisions, Dr. W., my plastic surgeon, did extensive grafting to correct areas of tight shallow skin. A twilight-sleep type of anesthetic gave me the sensation of falling asleep but never escaping the operating theater. I heard voices around me, people were cutting and sewing, but I remained amazingly indifferent to all of it. Now seeing both Walt and Steve, being told I was to stay in the hospital another day, and discovering an IV tube dangling next to me, I began to realize this was more than the brief outpatient surgery with which I was familiar.

"We were told that you would be yellow," said Steve, continuing to be jovial, "but you don't look any different."

"That's good," I replied.

"They told us the yellow pigment was a test to make sure the graft had circulation in it," explained Walt.

I returned home the next afternoon with new incisions on top of old scars and fresh cuts into new territory accomplishing a graft. How many stitches? There were so many that no one had attempted to count them. In ten days I would return to the clinic to have them removed.

Easter came while I still had my stitches. What echoed for me in the sacred text were the words of doubting Thomas, who vowed he would not believe the Resurrection account until he could actually see the nail prints on the hands and the wound in the side of the Crucified One, now said to have arisen. *Come, see the marks of the nails,* said the Lord speaking to Thomas, *and the wound in my side. Do not be disbelieving.*

The resurrected Jesus had retained his scars! His glorified body, now prepared for the throne of heaven, bore the scars and sufferings of earth. I thought long about scars. His scars identified him as the Savior of the World. My scars . . . they too were my identity. Suffering is cheapened when labeled as meaningless or just "tough luck." Wisdom has deepened for me, character strengthened; thus far I give all my crises credence.

When the ten days were up, I returned to Dr. W. with an absurd question. Knowing him to be a Christian and that Easter was still alive for us, I took my chances.

Always greeting me with the smile I looked forward to, he brushed aside the white gown that was thrust over me as I sat in the big adjustable chair. He probed his previous work with an experienced eye and finally said, "It's healing well. Let's get rid of the stitches."

I leaped in with my question just as he was turning me over to Nurse S., who was standing by with snipper and tweezers.

"Dr. W., do you think my resurrected body will retain all the scars you have so skillfully created?"

He gave me a puzzled look and I hastened to say, "I'm not being facetious. I'm quite serious."

Hiding his astonishment with a cliché, he replied, "Only what's done for Christ will last."

I wished he had said more. Maybe it had never occurred to him that his artistry might have implications for eternity. I could understand, too, why he might laugh.

I returned to my oncologist for a checkup in late July with the hope that the new hormone I had been taking was being effective. I had discovered no new nodules and felt confident. Dr. H. was pleased regarding the all-important x-ray. "Remember, last time we found the beginnings of lung involvement again? Now all this seems fainter; it's stabilizing. I'll have you return in four months." As usual he dismissed me with a pat on the shoulder. "You're doing great."

Another reprieve—four months before I needed to worry. This has been the story of my life. For years people have been telling me, "With your attitude and your positive thinking, you are winning your battle." I always welcome this statement and take it only as a compliment, never sure that it is altogether true.

I am thinking about hope these days even as I thought about scars. Hope cannot be defined simply as optimism, positive thinking, or unswerving mind set. If this were true, then would the many people I've known who died of cancer have lived if they had thought more positively? Hardly. I remembered Elizabeth Hofter, the woman from Germany, who shared my room back in 1981. She died two years later; her husband sent me her death notice and thanked me for being her friend while in the Rochester hospital. Not only did she have hope, she instilled it in her family and others like me. Or Kathy, one of my students stricken with leukemia, whom I remember with fondness as she played her guitar for ballads in my English class; her enthusiasm for life could only be called hope. Then there was Aasulv, a Norwegian colleague from our Africa years, who with his wife stayed with us while he sought help at the Mayo Clinic. He died soon after returning to Norway. He was, indeed, a person with hope who accomplished more than most of us in his lifetime. And more than all the others. I remembered Jan, who died of breast cancer, leaving a husband and four children. I had been spared the agony of leaving my half-grown son and my husband, years ago. She was taken, not because she lacked hope.

Neither is hope wishing. Hope is not merely imagining what we want or expecting miracles. Miracles are wonderful when they occur, but they do not come to all who pray for them. Wishing is the consumer in us, demanding a thousand wants and desires. Wishing has very little to do with hope.

Hope is personal. but it thrives in community with others. The friends I mentioned and I were bound together in hope for one another. Our hope always finds the neighbor and we are brought close because of it.

> Hope springs eternal in the human breast.
> Man never is but always to be blessed.
> —Alexander Pope.

How could I forget pondering those lines in English literature class? Hope is forward-looking, expecting a blessing, says Pope. Hope says yes to each new day and expects strength to live it, accepting all limitations. Someone has said that hope springs from hopelessness. It is the answer the human spirit gives to a lifetime of needs.

What thoughts do I have about the eternal hope of Christians? Since we mortals will experience only an infinitesimal part of the time and space of our present world, I am incapable of even imagining what is ahead for me. It is, however, the hope that undergirds all our hopes: trusting the ultimate goodness of our Creator.

I am reminded of one of Pastor T.'s frequent visits when I told him a dream I had the night before. "It was getting dark as I walked along a familiar trail in the woods near my old home. I stopped in fascination at a place where an animal, perhaps a deer, must have lain. The long grass was lodged, and at one end was a slight rise that resembled a pillow. Fatigue such as I have never experienced before came over me. I wanted more than anything else to lie down in this bed on the ground! I knelt to do so when I woke."

He smiled. "Nice dream—have you thought what it might mean?"

"No, that's what I would like to ask you."

"There are two things here, extreme weariness—and a place to lie down, what might you make of that?"

I answered bluntly. "I think this symbolizes the

grave! It was a place of peace. I only wanted to sleep on the earth I had grown to love and respect."

"I think we all look forward to eternal rest even though we aren't aware of it," he continued, expecting more from me.

"My unconscious is telling me I am weary and ready for sleep. I guess that is it. What can you tell me about eternal hope now that I am ready for sleep?"

"Joy comes in the morning!"

About the Author

Margaret Christlock Gilseth was born March 31, 1919, in Wanamingo, Minnesota. She graduated from Augsburg College, Minneapolis, Minnesota, with majors in English and history and credentials to teach in secondary schools. She did graduate study at the University of Washington. In 1964, she earned a Master of Arts degree from the Lutheran School of Theology at Chicago. She taught for twenty-five years in secondary schools in Minnesota, South Dakota, and Washington. She and her husband taught four years at Marangu Teacher Training College in Tanzania, Africa. She presently lives in St. Charles, Minnesota.

In November 1987, Askeladd Press published her first novel, *Julia's Children.* A second book, *Fjord Magic: Getting Acquainted with Norway*, a nonfiction book for young readers, came out in 1989. She has published two collections of poetry, *Rainwater* and *Christmas Wreaths.*

She received the Distinguished Alumna Award from Augsburg College in October of 1993.

She is grateful to Theresa Haynes and Ann Brownwell for their invaluable help in editing the original manuscript of *Silver Linings: Living with Cancer.*